FINDING A BREAK
IN THE CLOUDS

A Gentle Guide and Companion for
Breaking Free From an Eating Disorder

By

Kyrai Eya Ann Antares

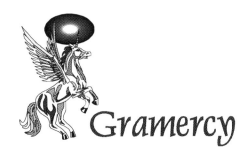

Gramercy

COVER PHOTO BY CHARLIE RED CLAW

Order this book online at www.trafford.com
or email orders@trafford.com

Most Trafford titles are also available at major online book retailers.

Print information available on the last page.

ISBN: 978-1-5521-2676-9 (sc)
ISBN: 978-1-4122-4313-1 (e)

Trafford rev 12/04/2019

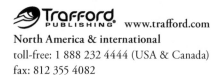

www.trafford.com

North America & international
toll-free: 1 888 232 4444 (USA & Canada)
fax: 812 355 4082

This book is for:
Christine,
and the young women and men I had the privilege of learning from and
sharing with at the Beaumont Hospital eating disorder support groups.
Thank you.

Acknowledgements

I would like to express my deepest gratitude and appreciation to the following miracles in my life. Without them, not only would this book not be possible, but I would not be the woman I am today. We are all in this life together, finding our way home. We need each other. We help each other. We teach each other. Thank you for being a part of my life experience.

- My darling husband, my greatest teacher, and my best friend - *Joseph David Antares*. Thank you for your support in writing this book. It could not have happened without your help. From the first outline through the final draft, your comments, ideas, and suggestions have been priceless. You are the most talented writer I have ever read, and a superior, objective, honest editor. Thank you for helping me build Ivy and Kyrai. I love you. Thank you for finding me. Thank you for choosing me. Thank you for teaching me. Thank you for loving me. Just don't stop. Not ever.
- Chris Germain, Kevin Thompson, Carrie MacGillis, Kenny Germain. Thank you for all of your support through my times of trial - for going to the hospital with me, going to support group meetings, massaging my feet, listening to me complain, asking me about what was happening, and doing your best to understand. What a relief to go through all of this knowing that you would never give up on me. A lot of people don't have such a gift. Thank you for your suggestions, and for listening to all of my ideas as they sprouted from my mind. Thank you for never letting my struggle interfere with the strong and solid love that holds us together.
- Adam Germain. My dear brother, thank you for always believing in me. I feel very blessed that we have each other. We are the special ones! We have to stick together. I love you with all of my heart. Never stop reaching. Keep your eyes on the prize. *We can do anything - together.*
- Ann Rogaczewski. You taught me more than you could ever possibly realize. You gave me the opportunity to find silence within my self. In this silence I found the strength, perseverance, and compassion necessary to make this book, and so many other things, possible for me. My experience with you greatly deepened my relationship with God. Thank you with all of my heart and soul.
- John Rogaczewski. Thank you for never leaving me.
- The Royal Oak Beaumont Hospital eating disorders program. Specifically, Dr. Susan Gottlieb, Dr. Sakeyfio, and the many diverse, wonderful, miraculous people who attended the support groups. I would not be alive if I had never come to those meetings. Thank you for believing in me, listening to me, and encouraging my efforts in writing and speaking.
- Stefan Brink. From the first time we spoke, I knew you would alter my life completely. You started me on the road of natural foods cooking, physical healing, self-love, responsibility, maturity, and authenticity. I appreciate your presence in my life. Without your wisdom, gentleness, sincerity, and generosity, I would not be the woman I am today. I feel as though we have touched each other's hearts many

lifetimes over. Thank you for everything. Gabriella, thank you for the mothering you gave to me so sincerely, for the healing touch, and for being an example of delicious femininity. You inspired me to find the goddess within me.

- Jewel (Ambro), Sentia, Supriya, Tracy, Belle, Kriya, Ada, and Elisa. My sisters, the joy you bring to my life is indescribable. I feel so blessed to have such a warm, open, loving, supportive, real community of people to share my life with. I am thrilled that we have found a safe place where we can explore, share, create, sing, dance, laugh, grow, and become. I am very excited to see what happens next for all of us! **Jewel**, your innate magic is so obvious and delightful. What a relief it is that you exist! Just thinking of you makes me giggle. You see me. I see you. I love our perfect friendship that bends and grows with the gentle breeze of life. You are intensely dear to me. I love our devotional connection. I love how you love God. Thank you for being alive. **Sentia**, my sister. We have built a family of love. Thank you for the mirrors, the love, the songs, the fun, the shared tears, and the mutual encouragement and admiration that I value more than words can say. Thanks for sharing clothes with me, talking to me about **everything**, and for exploring the depths of sisterhood. **Supriya**, you have had an immense impact on my life. Without you, I would never have begun the path of breaking free from illusion. I look up to you, and I honor our deep connection. Thank you for bringing Amma into my life. Thank you for your support in all of my diverse endeavors. **Tracy**, thank you for teaching me about myself. Thank you for giving me feedback during the beginning stages of this book. Let's break free together! I am so proud of you sister. **Belle**, you bright shining star child! Keep reaching! Keep asking! Keep rising! You are on your way. Thank you for appreciating me, and for your ongoing encouragement. **Kriya mama**! You are quite an inspiration. Thank you for encouraging my writing, and for reading the first draft of my intro. You are such a gift to all of us. **Ada**, thank you for valuing me, for believing in me, and for staying in touch! **Elisa**, even when we aren't in touch for awhile, I feel our friendship in my heart. Thanks for listening to me, talking with me, and laughing with me. I love you.
- Mike Buday, Edna and Gene Buday (Tasty Health gang). You are such wonderful people. Thank you for your interest in me, and in my book. Thank you for welcoming me into your family, and becoming my friends. Thank you for all of the encouragement, understanding, and appreciation.
- Melanie, thank you for opening your heart to me, and for trusting me enough to share your life with me. Thank you for being honest with me about your invader, and letting me try to help you. We'll make it together!
- Brooklyn Paige Clendening, my darling friend from Meadowdale Street. You are so precious to me. Thank you for being such a pure example of God's love in my life. Thank you for believing in me, and for being my friend.
- Dawn and Darnell Branch, Ryan and Raydell, Thank you for teaching me about true love and friendship. Dawn, I hope you know that even when we don't talk often, I think of you every day, and I know you are in God's hands. You have such a beautiful family. Thank you for taking me into your heart. I will never forget our time living together at Olivet. I still get chills whenever I remember your singing. I love you,

sister. Ryan, you are pure joy to me. I think of you all the time. Thank you for being such a precious, special little angel. I love you.

- Carlton Polk. Thank you for helping me learn how to love myself. Thank you for making me feel special. Thank you for never forgetting about me. Thank you for our beautiful memories from Olivet, and afterwards. You were always there, unconditionally, to listen, and to make me laugh. You are a dear friend to me. Thank you.

- Dr. Frederick Howell. Thank you for listening.

- Antje and Rob Carroll, Ethel, Deb Nevar, and Isabelle Flemming. Thank you for your continuous support through Magic Meal Express, and beyond. Your appreciation for my cooking kept me going on the challenging days.

- Also, Zen, Unkie, Vicki, Halina, Betty Draganski, Charlie Red Claw, Connie and Tom Leroy, Mary Ann King, Laura, Keith, Linda and Courtney, Cheryl and Pat, Mark and Stacy, Uncle Don, Auntie Alvira and Allen, Jack Arduin, Uncle Jerry and Auntie Joyce, Beata Jackowska, Mike Demko, the Self Esteem Shop crew, Carey, John, Crystal, Oliver, Bill, James Law, Brian, Leslie, Sarah, Lisa, Leslie Wood, Ken and Angela Germain, Bianca, Harrison, Swan, the Fruit Cellar crew, Marco, Jodi, Billy, Nick Ciantar, Bruce Merritt, Adrian, Gwennie, Ashley, Chris, Katherine, Chantel and Dave, Jason Reed, Skip, Justin, Nicki, John from Oz, Lliam, Rob Woollard, Marc, Sara and David Woollard, and Ron and August Gentry. Thank you for the unique and wonderful ways in which you touched my heart and supported me over the years. I have learned valuable life lessons from all of you, and I am thankful that our paths have intertwined.

- Ammachi. Divine Mother, how can I ever thank you enough. May my entire life be dedicated to you. Every breath, every word, every action. And may that begin to represent the immense gratitude I feel in my heart. Thank you for my body. Thank you for this chance to awaken. Thank you for loving me. May I become what you would have me become. Dear God, thank you for my life. May it be used to serve you. The more I give to you, the more I seem to have. I feel so honored and lucky to be here. Thank you.

May we all live in gratitude.

Finding a Break In the Clouds

Outline of Contents

Chapter One: *WAR!* The first half of the author's intense personal story of surviving anorexia/bulimia. Intimately describes the psychological, emotional, and behavioral aspects of anorexia/bulimia.

Chapter Two: *Understanding the Invader.* Includes an explanation of the progression of eating disorders, a Declaration of War document, and an introduction to the idea of "the invader."

Chapter Three: *WAR! Part Two.* The continuation of the personal story of the author. Illustrates some physical repercussions of anorexia/bulimia, and the process of re-feeding.

Chapter Four: *Food: From Enemy To Ally.* Changing the idea of food from a feared opponent into appreciated medicine for the healing body.

Chapter Five: *Gentle Nutrition.* A new re-feeding plan which uses natural, unprocessed, and simple food as medicine.

Chapter Six: *What To Expect During Re-Feeding.* Prepares the reader for the physical, psychological, and emotional challenges of re-feeding. Includes activities and exercises to assist in times of struggle.

Chapter Seven: *Emotions: The Rescue Mission.* Reminds the reader that the natural emotional state is self-love, introduces the invader's thugs (Guilt and Shame) and the fear monster, assists in processing negative emotions, and reveals the secret weapon against the invader.

Chapter Eight: *The House of Being.* Expands the reader's idea of "self" to include more than the physical body.

Chapter Nine: *Recovery Insurance.* Many creative ideas for relapse prevention, including the creation of a Relapse Prevention Kit.

Chapter Ten: *Frequently Asked Questions.* Answers to questions commonly asked in support groups facilitated by the author.

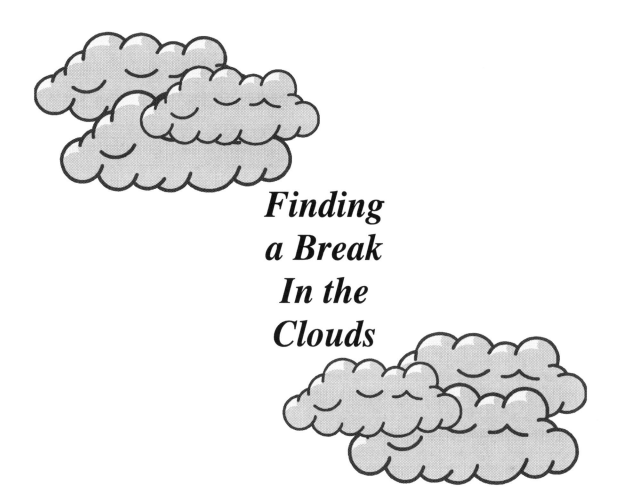

Finding a Break In the Clouds

The Self Esteem Shop

Spring, 1996. I needed self-esteem. I needed a job. What better place to work than the Self Esteem Shop?

This bookstore offered books, tapes, and CDs based on various areas of personal growth. Professional counseling tools and reference materials were also available. Carry, Elisa, and Lisa made working there an enjoyable and enriching experience. We spontaneously put on puppet shows for people shopping in the store. We did this in an attempt to lighten the atmosphere because many of the issues confronted there were serious and heavy. Puppets bring out the child self. The entire staff functioned more like a family than co-workers. Working there was a great way to ease my way back into society after being trapped in the cave of my eating disorder.

While working at the Self Esteem Shop I encountered people who were wrestling with food problems, or who were concerned about a loved one who was struggling. Books existed on the subject of eating disorders, some of which I recommended. But I found the resources to be lacking in one important way: there was nothing to help people deal with the daily obstacles/hindrances that make the challenge of recovery seem like too big a mountain to climb. I found no method available to help people understand how or why this disorder took over, or by what means they could reclaim their lives. I decided to create such a resource.

As I talked to people I could see that the wound from an eating disorder was especially difficult to heal because there was so much secrecy and shame involved. All of the issues which surfaced during a battle with anorexia or bulimia were incredibly personal and obscure. It became easier to let the world think it was just about the weight and oppressive media images. The tangled web of emotions and thoughts remained behind the scenes. The true causes of eating disorders were deeply rooted in the subconscious mind and damaged emotional self. It was like a huge confusing puzzle with only half of the pieces available. People were not used to talking about such raw and volatile issues.

Finding a Break In the Clouds is a gentle guide to accompany you through the depths of this intense process of recovery. It provides a nurturing and pliant structure within which you can rebuild your life. The ideas expressed are meant to inspire the discovery of your own secrets in relation to your eating disorder. Somewhere along the way you have forgotten what a miracle you are, and it is time to start remembering. Recovery can be wonderfully empowering because the work is personal. It is a battle fought for and by your self. No one knows this battlefield like you do. No one else can formulate your victory plan, and no one else will enjoy the benefits of cutting the controlling puppet strings of your disorder more than you. There are treasures available from this experience, and by owning the experience you gain access to the pot of gold at the end of the rainbow.

Anorexia and bulimia cannot be ignored. They are forces which must be reckoned with, and during this wrestling match within your brain and your heart, your soul is enriched in infinite and indescribable ways. Deciding to pull yourself out of the vortex of an eating disorder is not the end of one thing, but the beginning of many other things.

There is no manual to teach you how to begin living your own life instead of being imprisoned by an eating disorder. You must make your own. You must formulate an individualized mechanism *during* this process by using any tools available. Finding a Break In the Clouds may become one of your tools. The causes and deeper meanings of your experience are unique to you. There are some basic similarities among most cases, but the differences are as individual and diverse as human beings.

I have summarized my experience with anorexia and bulimia in Chapter One and Chapter Three for the purpose of identification - but this book is about you. Find yourself in these pages. Draw pictures and write poems in the margins. Take notes. There are no rules, no restrictions. This book is yours, this recovery process is yours, this life is yours. Take it!

CHAPTER ONE

WAR!

War was the perfect metaphor. War within myself. I was cut down the middle. Half of me wanted to recover, half wanted to die. The battle was continuous and exhausting. I fought my inner darkness four times, and each time was progressively more vicious.

Living In the Shadows

The first battle took place in high school. I was an active teenager who appeared normal and well adjusted, earning excellent grades and participating in school activities. Even though I seemed happy, I felt numb; no one knew me. Few people saw glimpses of my true self; she was far away most of the time, hiding in fear. Nothing I did, except chorus and tennis, was what I truly wanted to do. This was especially true of my relationships. I spent time with people who did not serve my best interest. One was abusive. Many were disempowering. I had chosen to be with people who did not believe in themselves or anyone else - including me.

When I was 15 years old I entered a relationship which quickly became abusive. The person I dated mentioned that my "fat stomach" would go away if I worked out regularly, so I began exercising at a gym every day. This was in addition to tennis practice five days per week. I followed a strict regimen of target muscle training and cardiovascular workouts approximately 2-3 hours per day. I quickly became addicted to over exercising. It produced a physical high, making me feel invincible and strong. I changed to a fat free diet, and started bringing my lunch to school to make sure it was absent of fat. I stopped eating desserts except on special occasions.

Peers noticed the change in my physical appearance, and I received praise for my efforts. I loved the attention. It made me feel special. Finally, I found an activity at which I could be the best. No one ever said anything about the dangers of exercising too much, or that fat was an important part of the diet. Everyone supported me, except my mother, who thought I spent too much time at the gym.

At this point, visible symptoms of the eating disorder surfaced. They were amenhorria (loss of periods), mood swings, and joint pain. The psychological symptoms, however, were far worse, and were not visible. I became more self-conscious, and obsessively compared myself to others. I thought everyone was prettier than I was, or wore better clothes, or had a flatter stomach. I thought that everyone was always staring at me and finding something wrong with me. I constantly worked at covering up my faults in order to feel that I was acceptable. The internal abuse was endless. If on special occasions I ate something with fat in it, I would beat myself mentally, until I could go to the gym and "work it off." I knew if I didn't make up for the extra I had eaten, I would be tortured by negative self-talk. It was like running from myself, but I always caught up and demanded more than I was giving. Nothing was ever good enough. The only time I felt happy was when I lost weight.

I used exercising to cope with life situations I was unable to face. I stopped talking to friends and family about my emotions, and turned instead to obsessive exercising. Because I only felt relieved after working out, I thought gaining control over my physical body was the key to happiness in my life.

My life was taking place on the surface of me. Nothing seemed to be functioning inside of me. My heart felt cold. My outer persona was the exact opposite of what I was feeling inside. I was being held hostage, while my eating disorder took over my life.

Temporary Relief

The first battle with my eating disorder ended when I went away to school at Olivet College. The new environment and distance from all that was familiar loaned me a sense of strength, which empowered me to end my abusive relationship and start over. The excitement distracted me from my exercise obsession.

I decreased the time I devoted to work outs, and became less strict with my food intake. I made new friends quickly, and felt more free than ever. Exercise, such as basketball and jogging, was more of a social activity than a requirement. Finally, I fit in somewhere.

One winter day in the cafeteria, I was walking to my seat carrying my tray of food. A friend said out loud, "Christine's getting thick!" He followed this comment by saying he meant it as a compliment, but he had already unlocked a door of self-abuse, which immediately flooded my mind. While he probably meant I looked healthy, I interpreted it to mean I was a big, fat pig; obese and out of control.

This ignited battle number two. Panic quickly set in. That day I began eating only lettuce.

My entire mood changed. I became serious and depressed. I slept more and spent less time out of my room. My mind was attacked constantly by self-defeating thoughts:
- I let myself go.
- How could I reverse all the work I had done?
- I am weak and out of control.
- I need to be strict now or I'll just become bigger and bigger.

After two weeks of the lettuce diet I ended up with the worst flu of my life. I had a high fever, dizziness, and I was coughing up yellow and brown mucus. I could barely walk. When my brother arrived to take me home, I was laying on my loft by the open window sweating and shivering. Some friends were trying to talk to me, but I could not understand them. A friend carried me to the car, and my brother drove me home.

My mom took me to the family doctor, and he said I had influenza caused by malnutrition. He asked if I had been dieting, and I told him I was only eating salads. He said I had to stop if I wanted to return to school. Still, no one mentioned the possibility of an eating disorder.

My mom left the room, and I asked the doctor if he thought I needed to lose weight. He looked at me and said, "Absolutely not. You look fine." I did not believe him. In my mind he was a part of the big conspiracy to make me overweight.

I wanted to return to school, so I ate while I was home. I needed a new plan; a way to make everyone think I was eating. The logical solution to my dilemma seemed to be purging.

When I went back to school, I began making myself throw up my food. At first, I didn't purge everything I ate; just anything with fat in it. It was difficult. My eyes watered, and my throat felt like it was going to burst. My neck muscles tightened, and my chest ached. I began favoring soft and smooth foods, because they were easier to regurgitate. The more I purged, the easier it became. In retrospect it seems frightening to me that my body actually adjusted to this harsh behavior.

My bulimia continued for a couple of months, and then tennis season began. I loved playing on the team, but it was a position which brought stress and pressure. The team was not strong, so I played number two singles and number one doubles as a freshman. I took my position seriously, and set high expectations. I burst into tears after most losses, and became depressed for days. My nerves were terrible, and I would sometimes have diarrhea before matches. I became more cynical and distant.

After a match in Kalamazoo the team went out to dinner at a fast food restaurant. I ate a fat free muffin, and went to the bathroom to throw up. At this point I could purge quietly and without watery eyes so no one would notice. This time, however, the toilet did not flush all the way. My best friend Dawn went into the stall after me, and saw my food. She approached me on the way out to the van, and asked me if I had been throwing up after meals. I lied and said I just didn't feel good that day, and usually didn't throw up. She said she hoped not. Lying became easier every day.

The Search for Acceptance

Toward the end of the school year I spent more weekends at home with my brother, watching his tennis tournaments with his college team. I began dating one of his teammates. At the end of the year I decided to come home and attend the same local community college as he and my brother.

My low self-esteem was temporarily raised due to my new relationship. I purged less; only when I ate something fattening, or if I felt I was too full. I thought if Mike loved me, I couldn't be so bad. My weight normalized and I was fairly healthy. This semi-relief period lasted about eight months. Then things began to change. Mike and I started drifting apart. I felt neglected and unloved, and decided there was something wrong with me.

This was the beginning of battle number three with my eating disorder. I started comparing myself to other girls. I talked constantly about losing weight. After months of hearing me constantly put myself down, Mike gave me a weight watchers book.

I was frozen with fear. My worst nightmare had just played out in reality. Not only was my own idea of being overweight verified, but the person I loved believed it too!

I immediately set rules:
   •no fat

•no animal products
•no desserts
•no eating after 6 p.m.

Soon the rules became more strict:
•only two meals per day
•drink only water
•no eating after five p.m..

Over the course of two months I dropped severely in weight. I received encouragement from Mike and his friends. They would compliment me, and ask me how I was losing weight.

"I eat less," was my practiced response.

People began commenting on my will power. I started to feel special; I was finally doing something right. Only my mom and my manager at work were concerned about my weight loss. When I was questioned I simply lied about what I ate.

At this time I was also singing in a rock band. There were three other girls in the group. We played in clubs on the average of once per week. This added more fuel to my disorder. I thought I had to be the thinnest one in the group. I was completely lost in vanity. I only cared about receiving attention and looking good.

I lost interest in talking about anything but food and dieting. I withdrew from friends and family. I even stopped taking college classes, because it was becoming more challenging to concentrate due to the lack of nutrition. I started working full time, so I would have more money to spend on clothes. The eating disorder made me feel successful, and led me to believe I did not need anything else. My value system changed drastically.

I began slowly separating from Mike, even after his attempts to repair the damage to our relationship. I became cold and unemotional. I rarely cried. I was sarcastic and shallow, preoccupied constantly with counting fat grams and recording my diet victories in my journal.

When Mike and I finally decided to end our relationship after two years, my sadness and grief barely showed. When I saw that he was upset, I acted upset; I did not know what else to do. I had become numb. My feelings were inaccessible, buried beneath a thick layer of my surface existence. The eating disorder became my coping mechanism. Instead of feeling something, I would distract myself with dieting. It seemed easier to hide from life rather than face it. I felt detached from the world. Everyone else lived there, and I lived nowhere. I was lost, sure that my strange, secret friend was all I had to hang onto.

Unhealthy Coping

Trapped in the cycle of anorexia, I became more restrictive every time I felt unhappy. I started spending time walking around health food stores and reading cookbooks. I obtained a new job at a health club, so I could start exercising in order to lose more weight.

Physical signs of damage began to surface. My arms and legs fell asleep at night, and I was bleeding when I had bowel movements. I also experienced several illnesses due to weakened immune function. I went through repeated bouts of strep throat, upper respiratory infections, sinus infections, flu, colds, and eventually mononucleosis. I was also experiencing much pain in the reproductive organs from endometriosis.

My energy was extremely low. I found everything exhausting. I avoided activities I once enjoyed. I quit the band I was in, and spent more time alone, working out, or shopping for clothes. I was afraid of spare time. I thought that if I wasn't doing something constantly I would eat. My mind would torture me for days, until I equaled it out with extended exercise sessions or less food. Every activity had the purpose of distracting me from eating. At night I wrote in my journal about what I ate that day and my goal for tomorrow. I was a walking dead person. Emotionless. Empty. The war raged within me. The eating disorder was winning. It was relentless. It was never pleased. It wanted complete surrender.

Pulled Out of the Cage

I met a fitness trainer at work one day, and I asked him if he could help me become leaner. We met for a training session during which he told me I did not have an extra ounce of weight on my body. Of course I did not believe him.

Two weeks later he asked me out on a date. At this point I was full of self-doubt and insecurity. I was nervous around him, and never knew what to say. My fascination with my world of dieting had impaired my ability to interact socially. I felt stupid. I did not know how to talk. I stuttered sometimes. I was no longer fluent in conversation. I felt surprised that Rob was interested in me. He kept asking me out, and I kept going. I felt detached. I was watching myself, like a shadow following its body around - but not actually participating. As we spent more time together my shell began to crack. I fed off of external validation from his compliments and attention. This caused something in me to shift. I started half-believing that I might be lovable.

Rob counseled me on nutrition. He told me how much I should be eating each day. I thought he was crazy at first, it seemed like so much food. He told me I should incorporate more grains and vegetable protein into my nutritional program. I had become completely vegetarian. I experimented with cooking by making dinners for Rob. He loved to eat, so it worked. Slowly, I ate more.

I did not know I had an eating disorder, and I was obliviously going through the re-feeding process with Rob as my coach. I experienced all of the uncomfortable symptoms such as:

- gas
- bloating
- nausea
- headaches
- stomach cramps
- sleep problems
- energy fluctuations

I eventually reached a healthy weight, and was exercising at a normal rate. I saw myself through Rob's eyes, and he loved me. I felt better about myself. But I soon learned that self-esteem from an external source and not rooted in myself, could never last.

In April of 1995 Rob and I took a trip to Arizona. On that trip Rob began to act differently. His energy level dropped, and his mood was unpredictable. After the trip Rob's health became worse, and he was diagnosed first with mononucleosis, then depression, then chronic fatigue syndrome.

I couldn't figure out what I had done wrong. I immediately felt like a failure. Everything was my fault. I weighed myself for the first time in months, and was shocked at the amount of weight I had gained. The demon was back. Battle number four.

The Invader Reclaims Territory

Anorexia and bulimia began a hostile takeover. I immediately implemented restrictions. I worked out more, ate less, and started to lose again. I drank coffee for energy. I purged anything of substance. This was the first time I participated in both anorexia and bulimia simultaneously. The struggle was full force this time. The terrible thoughts came back worse than ever, punishing me for "letting myself go, getting out of control, losing will power." I labeled myself a complete failure; I had lost everything of value.

The weight dropped faster and fell lower than it had in the past three battles. Rules were more strict. I ended up eating only a bowl of fruit in the morning and a plate of steamed vegetables for dinner. Water was the only liquid I ingested, except for a treat of apple juice once a week - if I was "good." I read an article which stated that drinking water contributed to weight loss. I increased my water intake enormously.

At this point I was attending The University of Michigan-Dearborn, part time. I secluded myself, and studied constantly. School was a way to take my mind off food. It was difficult, though. My mind would wander in the middle of class to thoughts of how many hours it had been since I ate, or what vegetables I would eat for dinner. I compared myself to everyone around me. I was constantly nervous and afraid that I looked stupid or ugly. I carefully chose my clothes each morning, and meticulously applied my make up. If people were eating chips and soda in class, I would pride myself in having the will power to resist.

People whispered about me in class. People stared at me in the hallways. Once I heard a classmate say, "Oh my God, look how skinny that girl is!" Every comment became fuel for the disorder. I loved and hated the attention at the same time. I longed to be normal, but feared being like everyone else.

My eating disorder convinced me that restriction was the only way to cope with emotion. It left me unable to make decisions in my life. I stopped living. I stopped feeling. I was at the beck and call of the eating disorder's will. It was victorious over the part of me who wanted to live. I was a prisoner. I was paralyzed with fear.

A Prison of My Own Making

Then something changed. I could see that I no longer had a choice. The option of eating no longer existed. I was not allowed to change my mind, and I thought I was insane. I realized that my life consisted of active weight loss and feeling righteous because of my will power. I could not think of anything else, even if I tried. Studying was extremely difficult, because I would find myself thinking about fat grams or how much water I was consuming. I stared off into space. When people talked to me I nodded, but had no idea what they were talking about. I was more tired than ever, and only had enough energy to go to school and come home.

Thoughts of asking for help crossed my mind, but were quickly shot down by the idea of having to gain weight. Besides, I was sure my family would put me in a mental hospital, if they knew what I was thinking all the time. Normal life was no longer a possibility for me. I only had enough energy to be anorexic - so that was all I did.

Through losing weight I thought I was fixing myself, but I was making everything worse. No amount of weight loss could heal the emptiness inside my heart. All my life I thought if I had the right boyfriend, the right clothes, the right friends, the right job, the right major in school, that it would make me "okay."

The End of the Rope

One Sunday morning in May of 1995 I was seated at the dining room table, studying for my final in Russian history. My mom and Kevin, her boyfriend, came into the room to eat breakfast. I went into the kitchen, filled my coffee cup, and returned to the table. My mom looked at me.
"Have you been losing weight?"
"Maybe a little," I said.
"How much more weight do you think you need to lose?" she asked, obviously alarmed.
"Just five more pounds," I stammered.
In making that statement I saw clearly for the first time that I had been saying "Just five more pounds" for months, and that those five pounds were never enough. 10, 20, 30, even 40 pounds later my eating disorder was still not satisfied.

I burst into tears. A true part of me was finally able to show. Fear, anguish, anxiety, and confusion poured out of me that morning. After years of hiding my dark secret, after endless self-inflicted punishments, after enduring a continuous six-year battle - I asked for help.

I told them everything. I told them I was out of control and that I *couldn't* eat, even when I wanted to. I told them I was constantly cold and depressed, and did not know what to do. My mom felt shocked and scared. She had not noticed the full extent of my weight loss or restrictive behavior.

It was as if an alarm went off. The world stopped. Nothing was ever the same in our house again. My sister immediately gathered all available information on eating disorders. We started reading, and found a support group at Beaumont Hospital in Royal Oak, Michigan.

It made me feel uncomfortable to place the phone call to find out the meeting days and times. It was the first time I had to talk to someone as if I were an "anorexic." In my mind, I knew something was wrong, but it was not anorexia. It had to be something else. Going to the meeting was simply a way of proving that fact. I didn't have any major health problems, and I wasn't *that* thin. The idea of anorexia or bulimia seemed impossible. They were the diseases featured on talk shows; not in my life. I had never thought of eating disorders as just *happening,* without the person being aware of the progression.

Naming It

That Monday I drove to my first meeting. My body was tense and my mind was racing. I don't know if I was more afraid of having an eating disorder, or of not having one. Either outcome seemed overwhelming. Fear filled my brain. I was sure I would be the fattest person at the meeting, and everyone would think I did not belong there. I thought they might ask me to leave. I decided I would not talk during the meeting. I just wanted to listen to everyone else. I found the meeting room, walked in, and sat down as quickly as possible.

Three women were there. I immediately began comparing myself to them. One woman was drinking diet soda. I said to myself, "See, I'm not anorexic, I only drink water. I don't even like diet soda."

A few more girls came in who were patients in the hospital program for eating disorders. The facilitator began the meeting. I was extremely nervous, and almost left. I thought everyone was staring at me, wondering why someone so overweight would be at this meeting.

I was relieved when the facilitator said that talking was not required. When she opened the meeting for people to begin sharing, there was an uncomfortable silence for a few moments - and then one woman spoke.

The first thing she shared was an explanation of why she was at the meeting, even though she was overweight. I was shocked. She didn't look overweight to me at all. She said she had just had a baby ten weeks prior, and was trying to lose the weight she had gained during pregnancy. She had gone through eating disorder phases since she was in junior high school. At this point she was alternating between eating one day and then fasting four days. She said that she had passed out a couple of times, and that she had decided to try to find help, so she could be a better mother for her baby. She said she was scared, and that the only time she felt happy and acceptable was when she was not eating. She said it made her feel high. I realized that was exactly how I felt when I didn't eat.

Another woman spoke about the voices inside of her head telling her not to eat. She said they were driving her crazy, and she couldn't live that way anymore. She was in the hospital. She said she wanted to recover, but she was afraid of gaining the weight.

I began thinking I belonged in this meeting after all. These women were describing exactly what I was experiencing. This little world I thought was unique to me actually existed in the lives of these women.

I continued listening with growing relief and growing fear. It was nice to know other people were going through the same thing I was, but I didn't want to have anorexia.

Toward the end of the group a young lady turned and looked right at me.

"Can you relate to any of this?" she said, as if she could read my mind.

I was terrified to say anything, so I just nodded and started to cry. The tears flowed like a river. My mind was moving so fast I couldn't make any sense. I felt like running out of the room. Everyone was looking at me, and my dark secret was exposed.

When the facilitator announced the end of the meeting, I darted from the room. The tears didn't slow down until I reached my car. I sat there in the parking lot, and realized my life had drastically changed in the course of one and a half hours. I was admitting I had an eating disorder; not only to those in the meeting - but to myself.

Part of me was terrified. Having a diagnosis changed everything. I would have to do something about it. I would have to attend meetings. I would have to learn more. I wasn't ready to let it go, yet. I didn't want to gain any weight. I did not want to face the world. I wanted to live inside of the world I could manage, the world I had created. I felt weak and deflated. I had deep feelings of failure. All that time I thought I had been doing the right thing.

Another part of me was relieved that I had someplace to go to talk about these things. I had thought no one else understood. I felt less secluded and less alone. I saw that I was not insane. A doorway began to emerge; a doorway which could possibly lead to freedom from this prison of mind.

I drove home and told my mom about the meeting. She shared in my half-scared, half-relieved feelings. I told her about a meeting for friends and family. My sister, my mom and I decided to attend.

The "family and friends" meeting was facilitated alternately by a doctor, nurse, psychologist, or nutritionist. It was quite informative regarding the physical effects of the disorder. My mom and sister were more afraid after the meeting, because they understood intellectually what I was putting my body through. A sense of urgency developed in them. It was clear that if recovery did not happen - death would.

The atmosphere in our house changed drastically. I felt exposed, as though I was walking around naked. My secret life had come to the surface. It was extremely uncomfortable. I felt territorial with my eating. I didn't want to answer questions about my habits. I lied to my mom when she asked me if I ever purged, because I wasn't ready to expose everything about what was happening. I wanted to maintain control over some things. I felt threatened, as though all my powers were being stripped away.

The eating disorder responded to this exposure by demanding more. I began thinking I was unworthy of being called an anorexic. I thought I wasn't thin enough to fit the diagnosis. One part of me turned the diagnosis into permission to dive deeper into the disorder.

Part of me felt special because of the attention I received from my family. I quickly latched onto the concern they displayed. I took it as a sign of love, and became dependent upon it. On days when I didn't believe I was receiving the adequate attention, I became depressed. I remember picturing my funeral, wondering who would show up and who would be crying. I fantasized about dying, about watching my funeral, and then coming back to life. On the days I did receive adequate attention, my mind would sometimes invalidate it by doubting its sincerity. My eating disorder had infested my emotions and intellect. That made negative, suspicious thoughts and feelings my automatic default position.

The internal war intensified. The eating disorder began functioning as if it were a living entity fighting for survival. My new awareness from the meetings caused it to attack. Because I was more aware of my behavior, the invader felt vulnerable and threatened. I realized that

9

all I cared about was food and losing weight. I had difficulty carrying on a conversation about much else. I began questioning the purpose of my life. I felt worthless. Was there no substance to my existence?

Flirting with Recovery

Due to the severity of my disorder and its rapid pace of advancement, my psychologist suggested a psychiatrist and a nutritionist who specialized in eating disorders. I had already decided I did not want to use anti-depressant medication for my depression. The psychiatrist suggested it, and I told him I saw depression as a normal state considering my circumstances. He sent me over to the nutritionist's office. She instructed me to begin writing down everything I ate. My weight was recorded at each visit. We talked about food and my relationship with my mother. I did not feel comfortable with her. I thought she just repeated what I said, and gave me no method to help me overcome my fear. My eating disorder had too much of an attitude for a passive approach to be effective.

I added little things to my food plan. I thought I would gain weight immediately when I added something, even one fig newton. I had no idea it would take more than that to begin reversing the momentum of the disorder. Also, I had become more active with running and drinking water, trying to balance out the added food. I was flirting with the idea of recovery, but not tackling it. My eating disorder even started adopting the habits other people would talk about during the meetings. I felt torn in half. I wanted to be free of anorexia, but was terrified of letting it go. I didn't want to lead such a small, limited life, but still fed off of comments about my thin appearance.

I knew what I was doing. That was the worst part. I could see how unhealthy it was to restrict and purge. My mind understood the medical ramifications I was learning about at the meetings. A wall stood between that understanding and its application to me. The confusion of that inner separation was difficult to describe. The eating disorder told me I was special because I had anorexia, and that without it I was nothing. Yet I was learning in the meetings and through reading that I was doing great harm to my body and psyche. Anorexia had become my identity. I did not know who I was without it. For five years food and exercise had been my way of coping with the world, because I did not feel strong enough to do it on my own.

I wanted to be well and not have to think about food constantly. But recovery seemed like a mountain too high to climb; an army too large to defeat. I wanted to be able to recover without gaining weight. I wanted to be free from the constant thoughts and anxiety, but did not want to go through the uncomfortable aspects of re-feeding. I procrastinated. I told myself I was not "that bad." I wanted proof that the eating disorder would kill me before I would give it up. I became obsessive about my health, and reported any sore throat, ache, or pain to anyone who would listen. I was searching for some physical sign that what the doctors were describing was actually happening to me. I thought if I could see I was nearing death, I could harvest enough strength from fear to push me through recovery.

The Deciding Factor

My fifth visit to the nutritionist was the first step in finding that part of me which had enough strength to fight the decisive battle and win the war. She informed me that I continued to lose weight because I was not adding enough food to my meal plan. She said if I did not stop losing weight and begin gaining at least one or two pounds, she would push for in-patient care at Beaumont Hospital.

I decided immediately that the hospital was not an option. I was terrified of eating animal products, and knew the hospital included them in the meals. I knew I would have absolutely no control in that environment, which scared me even more than re-feeding. I realized if I recovered at home, I would at least have control over my food choices. I drove home from the appointment, and made a piece of toast. I spread one teaspoon of peanut butter on it - and made myself eat it. The whole time I reminded myself that it was this, or the hospital. I decided to eat toast and peanut butter once every day, and incorporate a few more suggestions from the nutritionist.

My mom and I went shopping at the health food store, and tried to compromise on food choices. I wanted everything fat free, and she wanted everything normal. We found a compromise on most products. It was difficult. I knew she only wanted me to be healthy, but she could not hear the voices invading my head every time I picked up an "unsafe" food and put it in the cart. It was torture. Even though this situation was filled with struggle, it became clear that an intense love was the underlying force in my mom's concern.

Over the next couple weeks I added food to my meal plan. I gradually incorporated more grains in the form of toast, bagels, cereal, and sometimes pasta. I also added snacks of fruit or fig bars.

Eating was hard work. The most difficult times were after meals. I thought I could feel fat growing on my legs. I was sure my pants would not fit in the morning. I was convinced that everyone would notice how big I looked after every meal. I thought everyone would start talking about how much weight I was gaining. But I kept eating, watching anxiously for the light at the end of the tunnel.

My body was run down from all I had put it through. My joints ached and my arms often fell asleep. I also experienced chest pain and difficulty concentrating. Feeling sick and tired made recovery seem more difficult, but it also motivated me. I knew the only way I would ever feel physically better was by eating.

I continued to regularly attend the support group meetings on Mondays and Wednesdays. They were a strong force in my recovery. I was able to ask questions about the feelings of discomfort I experienced during re-feeding.

After deciding to recover I became somewhat paranoid about my health and survival. I was afraid the damage to my body was permanent, and that I would die before I could recover. I started to take note of every physical ailment. I reported swollen glands, sore throats, headaches, pains, nausea, and many other symptoms. Sometimes they were valid indicators of a virus or infection due to my impaired immune system, but sometimes they were simply results of my body's process of healing. I was on and off antibiotics several times, and seldom felt healthy.

During one meeting someone asked the doctor if a limb falling asleep had anything to do with her anorexia. My ears perked up because I had been experiencing this for months. He explained that every nerve cell was lined with fat, and if a person did not have enough fat

11

in the body, those nerve cells could no longer survive. This breaking down process led to the feeling of numbness and tingling. He said it was actually indicative of the beginning stages of nerve damage, and that some people actually lost the ability to move appendages due to this problem.

He also explained that centers in the brain slowly began to shut down due to lack of fuel. One by one the brain shut off its lights. This terrified me! I started to understand why I could not concentrate as easily as I once had been able to, and why I had to read things many times before understanding them. My brain was not fully functional. I asked if there was any way to retrieve the lost functioning. He assured me that with proper nutrition I could regain all that I had lost, as long as I was committed to recovery.

More Than My Disease

At another Wednesday meeting a young woman spoke about her recovery. It was refreshing to hear a success story. She told us how thankful she was to be done with anorexia, and how nice it was to have a life again. I envied her. I had such a long way to go before feeling normal or happy. My world seemed plagued with darkness. She said she regretted all the time she had wasted on dieting, because there was so much more to life. While she spoke, something in me snapped. I realized I had nothing to talk about except food and dieting. My *health* condition had become my *life* condition. When people asked me what I had been doing for the last couple of years, the most vivid memories were my weight loss victories. This was no longer enough for me. I wanted to *be* something more than my disease.

I decided to make a list of all the things my eating disorder was preventing me from accomplishing. Graduating from college, playing tennis, adopting a dog, singing in a band again, flying a kite, walking, camping, being with friends and enjoying it, writing, learning, obtaining a job, and feeling normal. This exercise was helpful because it transformed, in my head, my eating disorder from a roadway into a roadblock. It went from being the sense of control I had taken it to be, to being exposed as the parasite it truly was. I clearly saw how anorexia had marched in and overthrown my will to live.

On the days when eating was a challenge, it helped to review my list of what the eating disorder prevented me from achieving. It brought my motivation to the front of my mind. It served as ammunition to fire at the negative and defeating thoughts sent by the eating disorder. Even though I did not want to eat at times, and I felt like I was under a dark cloud of confusion, something inside knew I was going to be well one day, and that is what kept me going.

I wish I could describe the exact moment at which I felt confident about my decision to recover. However, the road was bumpy and winding. One day was difficult; the next easier. Slowly the difficult days became less frequent, and the easier days became more frequent. As I ate more I noticed the negative voices in my head were weakening. Eventually I faced less and less internal resistance to eating meals. My strongest ally was my desire to do something with my life.

After about four weeks into re-feeding I decided to look for a job. I chose a little health food store where I shopped often. I thought it would be a healthy and safe environment in which I could learn about healthy eating.

The Fruit Cellar was the first place I tested out telling people about my eating disorder. I started out by casually mentioning in conversation that I was trying to gain some weight. I was surprised at how many people expressed relief that gaining weight was my goal. Many people said they had been worried about me because of my appearance. Telling people helped me to erase some of the shame involved in having anorexia and bulimia. I began to see that shame was just a trick played on me by the disorder, to keep me from exposing it. Talking with people also helped me see how distorted my body image was. I did not see my body the way everyone else did.

Work turned out to be a wonderful place to practice being out in the world again. My friend Marc would help me choose my lunch each day, and we would talk about many health issues. I felt loved and appreciated by everyone at the store. I even enjoyed a social life with some of the group. I started to see that life was not so bad after all.

CHAPTER TWO

Understanding The Invader

How Did This Happen?

How did life become nothing more than counting fat grams and calories? How did the goal of eating healthy turn into a paralyzing fear of food? How did self-alteration become self-destruction? How did this happen? This is an important question; one commonly asked by both those suffering from eating disorders, and by their families, who can also be affected.

The "invader" would like you to avoid answering this question. The very nature of the invader is to remain a secret. Staying just out of view is its specialty. It creeps in slowly, insidiously, stealing your secrets, and using them against you. By staying just out of reach, the invader maintains the illusion of an unsolvable puzzle. The more you know about the invader, the less power it has over you. Where light shines in, darkness disappears.

A helpful metaphor is home burglary. If someone broke into your home and stole your personal possessions, you would probably investigate. By finding out how the burglar entered the home, whether there was an open window, broken glass, or a loose board, you could remedy that problem, and take measures to prevent another break-in. You might buy some stronger locks, remember to lock windows, or strengthen the home's structure. The burglar would meet some resistance if another break-in was attempted.

Think of your body, personality, thoughts, emotions, and instincts as the home you live in. It is your energy field. The eating disorder has invaded your home. If you can track its progression and identify its point of entry, you can gain quite an advantage. You are no longer a helpless victim. The eating disorder is identified as something separate from you, which has "invaded" your being; not a permanent part of who you are.

Bridging the Gap

Understanding the invader is also useful in bridging the communication gap, between those struggling with eating disorders, and their loved ones. We are most afraid of what we don't know. If we don't know how this happened to our child, spouse, friend, or sibling, we may react out of fear. We may attempt to force a pace or method of recovery that makes *us* feel better. But it may not be the best plan for the person we are trying to help. Unless you have done it, it is difficult to understand why someone would restrict food intake to the point of self-starvation, why someone would throw up after eating, take laxatives, or use diuretics. Creating a step by step recount of the disorder's takeover gives friends and family a clearer view into this world.

The Infected Seed

I have found that almost every eating disorder can be tracked down to one fundamental, false belief. This one belief becomes the basis for a myriad of self-abuse patterns. It keeps people in the cycle of underestimating their greatness.

This false belief is:

There Is Something Wrong With Me!

Something happens during life's early stages, which plants this infected seed in the garden of your psyche, and you believe it! Perhaps it is something someone says to you when you are a toddler. Perhaps it is lack of affection during infancy. Every time something happens which hurts your feelings, makes you feel inadequate, unacceptable, or unlovable, you pile it on top of that infected seed. A pile of every hurtful incident collects and turns into fertilizer for the infected seed. The infected seed grows into a plant with gnarly vines and prickly thorns, and starts strangling all of the other plants in the garden. Soon it is so entangled with the rest of your life, you think it is a part of your true self, when it is only an overgrown lie. As this lie creeps its way into your thoughts, it causes you to begin searching for a way to "fix" yourself - and the invader (the eating disorder) shows up wearing the mask of a friend, promising to solve your every problem. But behind that mask is a parasite; one ready to suck the life out of you.

The Progression

I see eating disorders as occurring in four phases. Keep in mind that these phases occur in their own time. You may experience any given phase for a week, a year, or 10 years. You may not even reach phase four. You may experience bits and pieces of each phase. Each story is unique.

PHASE 1: Phantom Bliss

In the beginning, the eating disorder actually appears as a solution. A mound of heavy, dense, dark energy has become part of the self-concept. It is like a wild, raging river being held by a weakening dam. There is a feeling that it has to come out some way or implosion may occur. You start looking for some method of relief. The search for a toxic emotion processor begins.

For a future alcoholic the "solution" may come when someone offers the first drink. The alcohol induces a state within which problems seem to dissipate, and the person finally feels free from insecurity and self-loathing. For an anorexic or bulimic, the relief would be found in dieting, exercising, taking laxatives, purging, or using diuretics. For me, the moment of relief came when the person I dated in high school suggested I start doing sit-ups for my "fat stomach." I started working out. Soon I was over-exercising. His comments provided a channel through which the built up darkness inside of me could finally come out. Many would argue that his comments were what planted the seed of disorder. I disagree. I believe that if the original belief (there was something wrong with me) had not been present, I would not have listened to his comment, and would have found someone healthier to spend time with.

During the first phase of the takeover, the invader is in the back ground watching. It is learning about your weaknesses, letting you feel the high of not eating, over-exercising, or bingeing and purging. It lets you think you have found the answer to all your problems. It lets you soak in the compliments from people, which make you think you finally found an activity in which you can excel. It lets you feel a much needed sense of control over your life. You may start wondering why you hadn't done this sooner. Everything seems more manageable. The gratification from seeing results in the form of weight loss elevates you. You are on top of the world. A success. Finally fixing all that is wrong with you. Little do you know the invader is lurking in the shadows - waiting for the perfect time to strike.

PHASE 2: Taking Prisoners

The invader has listened to you cheer yourself on during phase one, and has learned to imitate your voice. It starts telling you there is a way to feel even better. There is a way to fix even more of your problems. You can lose more weight, and lose it faster. There has to be more bliss where this came from.

The invader then begins to take prisoners. The first prisoner is the emotions. Emotions are a potent force. They fuel all action, both detrimental and beneficial. The invader lures you in with a flourish of positive, intoxicating emotions. While you are distracted by this temporary euphoria, it collects your overlooked negative emotions (fear, anger, jealousy, hate, guilt, shame) for later use against you. When you feel negative emotions, the invader convinces you that the only way to escape is the eating disorder behavior.

The second prisoner is the intellect. The invader starts urging the memorization of calories and fat grams. Your brain calculates constantly. How many hours between meals, what time is too late to eat, what foods are forbidden. The intellect sets the rules. The emotions enforce them.

Imprisoning the intellect allows for the capture of the third prisoner - your survival instincts. If your thoughts are overloaded with diet calculations, there is no time to stop and think about what long term effects might be waiting down the road. There is no mental energy available to assess the damage you may be incurring by restricting or bingeing and purging. Even if a friend or parent attempts to warn you of potential danger, your mind is racing during the entire conversation. Your innate survival instinct is over-ridden by constant mental activity. This is why obsessive compulsive disorder often accompanies eating disorders. If you are not constantly busy, you may have a moment to sit back and realize the extent to which you are destroying your life.

PHASE 3: Escalation of Force

It is during phase three that control over your eating disorder is lost, and the invader takes full reign. It brings out the full arsenal. It completely overtakes your inner voice, and converts it to a cruel instrument of self-torture. There are no more cheers for weight loss, only more demands. Purging only some of your food will no longer satisfy it, now you must purge everything. Two meals per day is too much, now only one is allowed. A whole package of laxatives is taken instead of just a few.

Paranoia begins. The invader labels everyone an enemy. Everyone is trying to make you fat. Everybody is lying about how you look. Restaurants can't be trusted. Friends can't be trusted. Family can't be trusted. Doctors can't be trusted. There is a global conspiracy to make you gain weight. You withdraw from people and avoid social situations, especially if food is involved. Everywhere you look someone or something is trying to trick you into eating. No one understands you. You are running from the voices.

The invader is screaming at you inside your head, saying things like:

- I am out of control.
- I am a big fat pig.
- I am not like everyone else, anything I eat will make me gain weight.
- I can only be happy if I lose more weight.
- I look bigger every day.
- I wish I didn't have a body.
- I shouldn't have eaten anything today.
- If I eat something I'll never be able to stop.
- I have to get rid of this food.
- I feel sick whenever I eat.

Distorted body image begins in phase three. If the invader can trick you into not seeing your weight loss, it will be easier to convince you to lose more. Something in the brain changes, and you no longer see your body as it actually appears. Strange desires begin to develop within you. You want to look sick. You enjoy it when people tell you that you look sick. Health becomes an undesirable state. To be healthy now means to be overweight.

You begin to feel protective of your disorder. You are suspicious of people questioning your methods. It is easier to be cold and unapproachable than to explain. When cornered, lying is the only option. The lies roll smoothly off your tongue, for you are defending what you now feel is your sovereignty. You feel completely alone, and you like it that way. The less distraction, the more time can be used for devising and carrying out further plans to lose weight. Your eating disorder is now your best friend. It is the only thing that can fix you, and now there seems to be even more to fix than when you first began.

PHASE 4: Drowning In the Lake of Pain

Phase four is the phase of insanity. You are now a slave to anorexia, bulimia, or both. You can no longer think for yourself.

EVEN IF YOU WANT TO EAT, YOU CAN'T!

EVEN IF YOU DON'T WANT TO BINGE AND PURGE, YOU MUST!

You no longer respond to logic. Completely irrational activities may emerge. You may be discovered exercising in the middle of the night. You may read cookbooks in your spare time. You may go to grocery stores, walk the aisles staring at food, and leave without buying anything. You may even purge liquids.

You have absolutely no faith in yourself. You believe you are a complete loser. You can't understand why it isn't working anymore. You are depressed. You feel worthless. You are miserable. **But you can't stop.**

You may want to ask for help, but the invader will not let you. You may know something is wrong, but the invader floods you with fear, and makes you believe if you tell anyone, they will think you are crazy, and ruin all the work you have done. It tells you that only you have these incessant thoughts about food. Only you have a hard time with concentration, or constant negative self-talk.

There is a distinct difference between phase three and phase four. Instead of feeling like you have to protect the invader because it is your savior, you believe you have to hide it because you are insane. You do not know who you are without your rituals and habits, which revolve around food. While you are completely miserable, you still have some illusion of control. You have become your eating disorder.

During phase four the invader goes in for the kill. Not only has it taken complete control over your emotions, thoughts, and behavior, it also kicks you while you're down. The darkest and most potent emotions, which were captured earlier, are now unveiled. The invader starts feeding you the most horrible, self-destructive thoughts imaginable:

- I do not deserve to live.
- I do not deserve food.
- By killing me, this disorder is putting me out of my misery.
- I am only a burden to everyone around me, they would be better off without me.
- Dying must be better than living like this.
- I am not worth saving.
- It is too late.

As this intense depression sets in, you may begin fantasizing about your funeral; wondering who would show up, who would cry. You may start making plans for your possessions, or for your children. You may feel impartial toward death, or curious about it.

Life has completely changed. You no longer have any interest in your goals, dreams, friends, or activities. You may not want to live this way, but you feel trapped by the invader. You feel incapable of swimming to the surface of the lake of pain.

JOURNAL BREAK: Making It Personal
Write or draw the progression of your disorder. Did you go through a phase that was not mentioned? Did you experience every phase described? How did the invader sneak into your life? What lies did it tell you? What self-defeating thoughts did it use to control you? What did it take away from you? How did it change your life?

Messages From the Bottom of the Lake of Pain

After someone has been consumed by anorexia, bulimia, or both, subtle cries for help may surface. These indirect signs may be sent from the subconscious mind in an attempt to survive the takeover. There is a force present which does not want to drown in this lake of pain.

Here are some obvious signs to watch for:

- leaving out a journal which describes disorder behavior
- leaving toilet unflushed
- mentioning weight or amount of weight loss

There are also less obvious messages:

- There could be a strong emotional reaction to contradicting and oppressive media images in relation to weight and physical appearance. There is a growing disapproval of society's obsession with physical appearance. On some level there may be self-directed anger about letting the invader in.
- Uncharacteristic emotional outbursts may occur, such as: unexpected temper tantrums, uncharacteristic weeping, or excessive laughter. This could be the unconscious mind bringing up a noticeable behavior that may inspire an inquiry from loved ones about what is wrong.
- There may be a noticeable disturbance when people talk about plans for dieting or weight they need to lose. Statements like, "You look fine the way you are, don't start dieting." Or, "It is who you are on the inside that counts." These are attempts to save others from the misery of the eating disorder.

Replacing the Out-dated Toxic Emotion Processor

The Toxic Emotion Processor is the mechanism through which you attempt to process the overload of stifled emotions which has accumulated inside of you. There are different kinds of Toxic Emotion Processors. Some are destructive, and some are healthy. Some work, some don't. Anorexia and bulimia are unhealthy coping mechanisms. They are inadequate methods for dealing with uncomfortable emotional states. But there are healthy replacements! There are ways to process toxic emotions in a productive and relieving way. Self-abuse is not the only way to live. You can retrain yourself to use healthy methods of emotional processing and release.

When the disorder started, restricting and purging seemed like good ways to reduce the over-load of toxic emotions. But this toxic emotion processor is now out-dated. It no longer serves you. It is damaging more than it is helping. It is holding you back instead of pushing you forward. It is an energy leak instead of an energy source.

JOURNAL BREAK: Healthy Coping
- What are some healthy things you could do to cope instead of restricting or bingeing and purging?

- Take a poll. Ask some friends and relatives what they do to process emotional energy.

You Are More Than This Disorder

After recognizing that this processor is no longer useful, it must be replaced. Begin by detaching yourself from the eating disorder.

ACTIVITY BREAK: Separate!
You can begin separating yourself from the invader by exposing it. It maintains control by letting you think that the self-defeating voice is your voice. By answering the following questions you can begin to identify the invader, and set it apart from your identity.

- When I see food, the voice of the eating disorder immediately tells me:

- When I do not eat, the voice of the invader cheers me on, saying:

- After eating, the invader attacks me with harsh thoughts, like:

- My eating disorder wants me to believe that without it I am:

■ The invader tells me that restricting or purging is the only way to deal with:

■ Expose the lie. Find a picture of your invader. This will give you an image to associate with your disorder; something to fight. It is no longer imaginary if you have a physical representation of it.

Perhaps, until now, you have been believing that all of these thoughts were yours. What if they were just a toxic system you temporarily bought into? What if these thoughts and beliefs have no permanent attachment to you, and you can choose not to believe them anymore? By peeling the invader off of your self-image, you have the opportunity to discard it, and release yourself from prison.

You can integrate the practice of exposing the lies of the disorder into your everyday life. During meals, say out loud everything the invader is telling you. Speak about the fears. Keep paper and a pen next to your plate, and write everything it is telling you. Scribble or draw out the fear and anxiety that surfaces. Do something active. Extract the invader from your mind, and it will lose power over you.

ACTIVITY BREAK: Who Are You?

Who are you if you are not just an anorexic or bulimic? Who will you be without these habits and rituals, which have been running your life? Many people do not know; and this creates fear, which causes a delay in commitment to recovery. How can you remember your true self, which has been imprisoned by your disorder?

Answer the following questions. They are meant to show you that parts of yourself have not been affected by the invader. They may lead you to a clearer understanding of who you are, and who you may become without the limitations of anorexia and bulimia.

• What is your favorite color?

• What kind of music do you like to listen to?

• Who do you think of as a hero?

- What causes do you believe in? Why?

- Describe, through writing or drawing, a peaceful place you would like to visit, real or imaginary.

- What is one of your biggest life goals?

- What is your favorite animal? Why?

- Write about or draw something you have always wanted to do.

- If you had one wish, what would you wish for?

Re-programming Your Brain

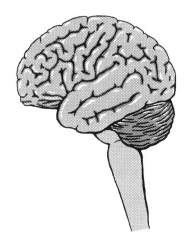

The brain is filled with billions of neurons. These neurons connect to form pathways. These pathways are memories. One pathway allows your brain to remember where the trash can is in your kitchen. Another pathway lets you remember the way to work. The only way to alter these pathways is to begin new ones to replace the old ideas. You must do something different in order to receive different results. For example: If you change the location of your kitchen trash can, it takes a couple days for you to stop going to the old location. In the brain, a new pathway which knows the new location is forming, and the old pathway, which is no longer useful, is beginning to break down. If a pathway is no longer used, it is broken down. You must do something different in order to see a different result. You must live in a different way in order to have a different life.

With this in mind, the formation of new neural networks to replace the useless ones, which support the eating disorder, is the physiological essence of recovery. You must start these new networks with the fundamental idea that nothing is wrong with you. Then the old pathways, based on the idea that something is wrong with you, will begin to break down. This is why the negative self-talk begins to lessen as health improves. The brain begins forming pathways which favor the feelings and sensations achieved from eating food. The more work put into recovery, through affirmations, consistency of eating, journaling, talking, reading, and listening, the more internal support is accumulated.

This is why it is important to say affirmations even if you don't believe them at first. (Especially if you don't believe them at first!) You are starting a new neural network. You are actually forming your brain cells into a new pattern to support self-care instead of self-destruction. It takes time and effort - but it is absolutely possible to teach your brain to send you positive messages.

MIRROR EXERCISE: Every morning when you wake up, and every night before you go to bed, look at yourself in the mirror and say one or more of the following:

- There is nothing wrong with you.
- I love you.
- I am proud of you.
- You are perfect just the way you are.

And while you're at it, wink at yourself!

After saying these things consistently for a couple of months, you will notice an urge to start adding some things. You may just begin to believe it! The purpose of this mirror exercise is to provide fuel for the part of you that wants to recover.

You Will Never Be the Same Again

The experience of developing, understanding, and recovering from an eating disorder is much too intense for you not to be completely altered and transformed by it. Even after complete recovery, you will not be the person you were before it started. Living the same way you lived before the eating disorder will only lead you back to its control. Here is the opportunity to create the life you want.

ACTIVITY BREAK: Make a Collage

Find some cardboard, wood, or poster board for the background of your collage. Gather some old magazines, a pair of scissors, and some glue or rubber cement.

During this entire activity try to think about your dreams and goals. Think about the person you want to become. Think about what life could be like without your eating disorder. As you look through the magazines, certain pictures will seem to light up or jump out at you. Cut them out and paste them any place on the board.

After completing your collage, write about how you felt, before, during, and after this activity.

SELF-CHECK

This exercise will be repeated throughout the book. When you see it, take a moment to sit quietly with yourself, thinking about how much of yourself you feel is controlled by the invader. In the image below, shade in the portion which is still under the reign of the invader. Choose the color and medium that feels appropriate. Then, in a different color, fill in the part of you which is free from the disorder. This tool may help you monitor how the eating disorder changes as you heal yourself.

If you like, replicate this figure and do this exercise every day. It may be a good indicator for what kind of day you are having. Start a self-check folder. On more challenging days, when the eating disorder seems to have more control, review self-checks from days on which you felt stronger and more capable of recovery.

Share your self-checks with your family and therapist. Sometimes pictures are an easier form of communication.

<u>SELF-CHECK</u>

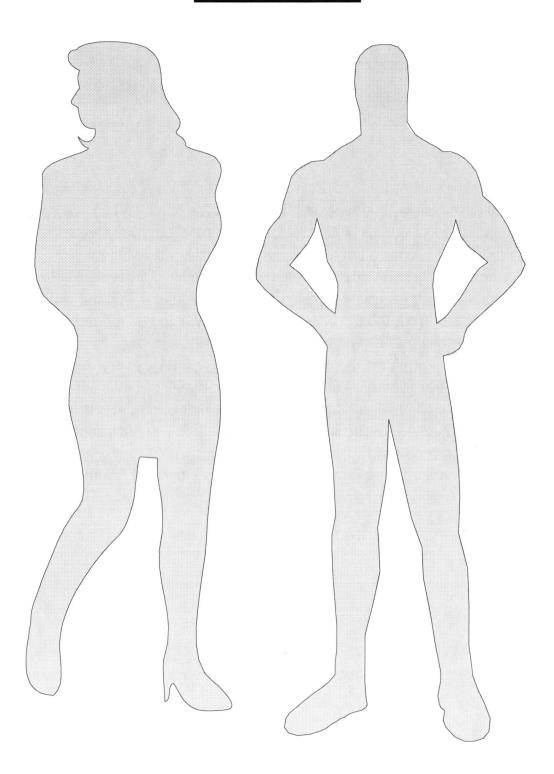

DECLARATION
OF
WAR

I,_____, hereby declare full scale war against the invader:_____(anorexia, bulimia, or both). Life conditions have become intolerable. I will no longer be held hostage by the negative self-talk, fear, and anxiety. I will no longer follow irrational and damaging rules of starvation or bingeing and purging. The invader is no longer welcome in my home.

I pledge to go to any lengths necessary to drive the invader out of this territory. I am committed to learning self-care, self-respect, and self-love I am deciding to take responsibility for my body. I am deciding to feed my body what it needs in order to survive. I am deciding to halt all persecution of my body; for it is an innocent victim of the invader's distorted reality. I am deciding to recognize food as an ally instead of an enemy.

I see the crookedness of the partnership I had engaged in with the invader. I learn from this experience and move forward. I see through the illusions. I am ready to fight the lies with a sword of truth.

In signing this document, I declare war on the invader. I commit to reclaiming my body, mind, and emotions. I agree to fight for my life against this force of darkness.

In signing this document, **I become a warrior, and I will stop at nothing short of complete and total victory!**

Signed: _____ Date: _____
Witness: _____ Date: _____

ACTIVITY BREAK: Build Your Warrior

It is important to empower that part of you which is capable of fighting the invader. You have a warrior inside you. You can tap into the power of your inner warrior by bringing that character to life. As you are more specific about the attributes of your warrior, your strength will be more available to you as you defeat the invader. Think of your favorite hero character. Is it a knight in armor fighting with a sword? A cowboy looking for a dual? An Olympic athlete ready for competition? A pirate setting sail for a new adventure? A black belt martial artist fully prepared for any opponent? An astronaut bravely exploring outer space? A monk impervious to all danger due to his/her deep faith and devotion? A tribal soldier surviving the primal danger of the jungle? An activist armed with passion and intellect? What represents strength and might to you? This is your warrior.

You can do this activity as a journal exercise, or as an art project. You could simply answer the questions and create your warrior in your mind, or you could actually create your warrior outfit and persona. It is up to you!

- What does your warrior look like? What does he/she wear? How big is your warrior? Does your warrior have a favorite weapon? Draw your warrior in the space below, or paste some warrior pictures from magazines and books, or go to a thrift shop and hunt for some warrior clothes. If there is a Renaissance festival in your area, you may be able to find some warrior garments there.

- What is your warrior's name?

- What are your warrior's special powers?

- Where is your warrior from?

CHAPTER THREE

WAR:
-PART TWO-

Physical Repercussions Emerge

Until the summer of 1995 I was under the impression I had no major health problems due to my disorder. I had no idea what damage had been incurred internally. The effects did not surface until I had already decided to recover, and began re-feeding. The small taste of a normal life I received from the first couple of months of recovery gave me the motivation to endure and overcome the challenges which were to arise.

During the month of July I began to experience back pain and discomfort in my left side. I thought it was a kidney infection, and when I was examined by my family doctor he agreed. Three days into the antibiotics the pain became worse. My doctor switched my medication, still treating it as an infection. Three days later I was feeling worse. Once again I went to the doctor, and he said a kidney stone might be obstructing the ureter, which would inhibit the kidney's ability to drain. He sent me to an imaging office where I was given an ultrasound of my kidney.

The doctor who reviewed my test explained that there was a blockage causing the kidney to swell and function poorly. He was not sure what the obstruction was, but recommended a procedure during which a stint would be placed in my ureter to allow drainage until the larger problem could be addressed. During this procedure a special x-ray called a retrograde pyelogram would be taken to help diagnose the source of the obstruction.

I called my mom, and she drove to the office so she could speak to the doctor and ask him some questions. After some discussion we both agreed to have the procedure done. I was not worried, for it sounded like a simple outpatient operation. I was worried though, about what they might find. Many things flew through my head. I did not want to lose my kidney at twenty years old. I had not considered a connection between this kidney problem and my eating disorder. I labeled it as bad luck, and began feeling sorry for myself. The depression became worse, and I felt less hopeful. In my mind, this was proof that I did not deserve to be happy like other people. I felt angry. I was trying to finally do the right thing, and another obstacle appeared. I continued to try eating more, but it seemed more difficult than before.

On the morning of the stint-placement surgery I noticed a change in myself. The other times I had gone through a procedure I enjoyed all of the attention. But this time when the nursed commented on my low blood pressure and my thin arms I felt uncomfortable. Something inside of me was shifting. What I once absorbed as sweet compliments were now leaving a bitter taste in my mouth. I was beginning to see that this was not the kind of attention I truly desired. While this was a positive change which motivated my recovery, it also motivated self-reproach. I was beginning to feel imprisoned rather than rescued by the small world I had created.

The doctor came back to see me after I signed the consent for anesthesia, and I was given a sedative. I began to drift off as they wheeled me down to the operating room. They lifted me onto another table, and strapped my arms down. They placed an oxygen mask over my mouth and nose, and instructed me to count backwards from 100. I was asleep by 99.

I woke up shaking and shivering. My entire body was convulsing. The nurses were piling warm blankets on me to try warming me. My teeth chattered and I felt sharp pains around the area of my kidney. A catheter had been inserted, which was uncomfortable. I was half asleep and half in an awakened panic. After about an hour my body warmed and I stopped shaking. Every deep breath I tried to take sent more pain through me.

My mom and sister helped me dress and wheeled me to the car. I winced from every bump on the road. The doctor said that this amount of pain was unusual. Under normal circumstances the stint did not cause this much discomfort. But due to my low weight, I had no padding to lessen the sensation.

Over the next few days I slept most of the time because of the pain medication. While awake, I tried to eat, but it was difficult, as I was in such pain.

The stint placement had been successful, and the problem had been found. The kidney had overgrown to twice the normal size in an attempt to accommodate the huge amounts of water I had been drinking. It would never reduce. Also, I had been born with a kink and a constriction in my ureter (the tube through which the kidney drains). Until this constriction was surgically corrected, the kidney would not be able to drain without a stint.

We met for a surgery consultation with the doctor who had done the stint placement. He seemed cold and unfeeling. He described the procedure which consisted of cutting me open from front to back, and cutting away a part of my kidney. I felt nauseous at the thought of being sliced open this way. I asked him how bad the scar would be, and he said I probably would not want to wear a bikini again. He said the recovery period would be 24 weeks. I was overwhelmed. My mom saw my heaviness, and asked that we have some time alone to discuss it.

I told her how sick I felt. I felt out of control. I was on a roller coaster which was moving too fast. I could not stop it. I had not anticipated the problem being so serious. I did not want to be cut open. When the doctor returned, we asked if we had any other treatment options. He spoke of a doctor who worked out of Henry Ford Hospital, who was said to have developed a progressive and less invasive procedure. He seemed skeptical of the doctor and the newness of the procedures, and was not sure if his approach was applicable to my condition. I asked for his name.

That afternoon I called Dr. Littleton's office and spoke to his secretary about setting an appointment. I had a hopeful feeling about him. Over the next week I collected all necessary x-rays and records for the appointment. I saw Dr. Littleton as my only chance of escaping that horrible surgery described by the first doctor.

My mom and I went to the appointment together. I felt nervous and anxious, hoping he would be able to help me. Dr. Littleton came in and went over my charts and x-rays, and then explained how he thought he could treat my situation. His procedure, which had a success rate of 85%, was performed almost entirely through a catheter with a scalpel and a tiny balloon on the end of a scope tube. The only scar would be from a drainage tube, and only about one inch long. This immediately felt like the best step to take. My mom and I asked him a few questions about the procedure, and told him about my eating disorder and my request for vegetarian food in the hospital. He advised me to gain as much weight as possible before the surgery. He recognized that my body was not strong enough for an operation. He would rather have waited for me to gain some weight. But the stint could only stay in for a relatively short period of time before it would stop working. I had about six weeks before the procedure. In the mean time I would have to undergo a series of pre-surgery tests. I left feeling hopeful.

I continued to slowly add food to my meal plan, and gained a little bit of weight. It was more challenging than I thought it would be. I thought I was eating tons of food and gaining weight quickly, but the scale showed just the opposite. The weight crept on slowly and gradually. I started to see that it was going to take a lot of time to reverse what I had done to my body.

Eating was a little bit easier after the discovery of my kidney problem, because something was actually happening as a consequence to my disordered behavior. I could no longer pretend nothing was wrong. The lies had been running my life. Stopping the lying was a long process. I also realized the more honest I was, and the more I tried to eat, the easier it became. I was still moody and angry a lot of the time. On my depressed days I felt worthless. I did not belong in this world. I often thought I was a burden to my family because of my health problems.

A Healing Current

The nature of recovery was part of what made it challenging for me. Slow and gradual and painstaking. I could not decide to recover, and then simply take some medicine. I had to diligently rework my thoughts, eating habits and emotions to align myself with a healing current. This was hard work every minute of every day, and it was exhausting. Many days I felt trapped between wanting to give up and feeling unable to complete the task. I felt ready to be normal and healthy, but had to go through the process to reach that place. I trudged on, through the bogs, marshes, and swamps. I did the work, even when I had a poor attitude toward it. "Complain as you will," I said to myself, "but eat!" With the development of my kidney problem came a fear which made me realize I could not go on that way forever. Either I would have to start doing the work, or I would eventually lose my life.

During this period everything seemed to revolve around my health issues. I felt buried by symptoms, tests, and doctor visits. My one relief came with the arrival of my 21st birthday. My sister and mom planned a surprise Hawaiian birthday party for me. A huge crowd of the most special people in my life came over to show support and love. It was wonderful. My sister even demanded that all of the food served be vegan in honor of my beliefs about humane treatment of animals. For this entire day I felt normal. I was reminded that life could be full of love and fun. The party reinforced the idea that family and friends were more important than how much I weighed. Suddenly I had a picture in my mind of what life might look like if I were healthy and able to function socially, emotionally, and physically. Even though it had only lasted one day, this experience motivated me through the rough road which lay ahead.

The Unexpected

On the day of my procedure, everything seemed consistent with the outpatient surgeries I had been through in the past. I had to be at the hospital early, fill out forms, have an I.V. started, and so on. My mom and sister came to the hospital with me. I spoke to the doctor before I was given any sedative, and he assured me that when I woke up I would not be in pain, because he had already ordered the pain medication that I requested. He said I would only have to be in the hospital for one day at the most. I would probably sleep the whole time. I drifted off feeling confident and relaxed.

An hour and a half later my own vomiting woke me up. My entire body was shaking. My teeth were chattering, and I was moaning and crying. Pain coursed through my body. It was as though I was being stabbed in the back and side. I rolled from side to side, trying desperately to find a comfortable position. Nurses were all around me, cleaning my vomit and trying to calm me down.

They had given me a different pain medication than the one I had requested. My body had rejected it, leaving me without pain relief. They told me they would have to order another pain medication from the pharmacy, and it would take an hour. Meanwhile, they were going to wheel me up to my room. My mom and sister were in the hallway when they brought me out. I was still crying and moaning and telling anyone who would listen how badly I was hurting. My sister became scared and started crying, asking why I was in so much pain. The nurses explained the mistake with the medication. My mom stayed with me until they brought the shot, trying to calm me down and help me feel better. But it was no use. I felt under attack. I had a tube sticking out of my back, a catheter inserted in my urethra, and an I.V. in my hand. It was hell.

After the shot of Toradyl was finally administered, the edge was taken off the pain. But it was still vicious. My doctor came to visit me, and apologized for the problem with medication. He also explained that my health was more fragile than he had originally thought. He had never seen someone in so much pain after one of these procedures. He thought it must have been due to my low weight and body fat. I had no padding around my organs. Also, because I was allergic to so many medications it was impossible to give me something stronger for the pain.

I wanted so badly to sleep, but could not find comfort. My mom read to me, and talked with me, and listened to me endlessly complain. The worst moments were in the night when she was not there. I just rolled around on the bed, waiting for morning. There was no relief from the pain. The doctors kept telling me to stand up and walk to encourage the healing process, but it was difficult to move, let alone walk. When forced, I would trudge slowly down the hallway, holding onto two people's arms, bent over and crying. I was quite a disagreeable patient. I was rude to the doctors and my room mate. I found fault with everything and everyone. I was constantly grumpy and crabby. Everything seemed too loud and too bright. I just wanted to crawl into a cocoon and sleep.

My first meal arrived on the day after my surgery. Pork chops and milk! I explained that I had spoken to my doctor, and was supposed to receive vegetarian meals. They knew nothing about that arrangement. I tried to drink some apple juice, and my body immediately threw it up. I was constantly nauseous. The doctors said I had developed sinusitis, which caused a nasal drip in the back of my throat. I could not keep any food down. After a few days of not eating anything, I knew I was losing weight. But for the first time in a long time losing weight was exactly what I *didn't* want. If gaining weight would take away any of that horrible pain, I was all for it.

On the fourth day of my hospital stay two psychiatrists came to visit. They knew of my eating disorder, and wanted to know why I was not eating. They thought I was trying to avoid recovery. I explained to them that at first I was given the wrong food, and then I was throwing up because of the sinusitis. They asked if I was purging. I became frustrated. They did not believe anything I told them. I was being treated like a typical, lying anorexic instead of a person. I again explained about the problem I was having keeping things down, and they asked me again why I was not eating. I began to cry. I could not express my thoughts due to the medication and my health in general. When I started crying they asked me if I thought my depression was worse, and if I was a danger to myself. They tried to write me a prescription for anti-depressants. For the first time I was actually wanting to heal, and they did not believe me. I told them that anyone in my situation would be depressed. I asked them to leave.

Just I Myself

This incident was important. It showed me that I wanted to recover more than I wanted anorexia. I no longer wanted to excel at having an eating disorder, I wanted to excel at being me. I was not typical, and did not want to be treated as such. The anger I felt toward the psychiatrists was packed with motivation and passion. I felt ready. I felt charged. Nothing was going to stop me. I was going to prove them wrong.

That night something happened that changed me even more. The doctors started to give me laxatives because I had not had a bowel movement since before the surgery. My stomach was bloated, and was not making any sounds. The laxatives were not working at first, and my blood pressure began to drop steadily. It was already low, and when it started to fall even further the doctors became concerned. They started doing different things to raise it. This continued for an hour or two, and I could feel tension in the room. I looked at my mom's face and knew she was afraid. It was after visiting hours, and she was not going anywhere. I became terrified. I thought I was going to die. I started to think about all the things I had not had a chance to experience yet. I thought about all the people I would never see again. I had no spiritual base to look to for strength. I had no idea what might happen if my body died. I realized I was not ready to go, and I prayed for another chance. I made up my mind to be committed to recovery. I wanted to live.

My blood pressure eventually turned around, and my digestive system began functioning again. My mom and I talked about how afraid we had been through the night. Something in me shifted strongly that day. I was afraid of death for the first time since my disorder started. Until this point I had been lost in thinking death would be better than life, which seemed too much to handle. Also, I had been convinced that everyone around me would be better off if I died, because of all the worry and stress I caused. But at that point everything seemed different. I saw that everyone, including me, wanted nothing more than for me to heal. Even though my body was weak and I had a long road ahead, my internal motivation was strong. I knew I could do it. I was ready to rescue the part of myself which was imprisoned by the disorder.

All of these realizations led to an important shift in perspective. I could differentiate myself from my disorder. I could see that the negative thought patterns which had been running my life were not *me;* they were coming from the disorder. I was its host and it was consuming me. It had tricked me into thinking I was just an eating disorder. This was a powerful insight. If this disorder was not me, but a cloak with which I had been hiding myself - then I could take it off! I could change it! I had a choice!

Fear accompanied this new step in recovery. I was not sure what I would uncover as I separated myself from this ominous cloak, which I thought had been concealing all of my imperfections. I had taken on the general identity of an anorexic/bulimic for so long that I no longer had a clear idea of who I was. Yet, for the first time I was certain that whatever I was about to reveal was going to be better than the dead end road I had been traveling.

Finally Home

After seven days in the hospital it was finally time to go home. It would take six weeks for my body to heal from the surgery, and then I would return and have the stint taken out. I was still in immense pain, and it took my every effort to sit up or walk. I felt fragile and weak. It was clear to me that I was responsible for my body's damaged state, and I was also going to have to take responsibility for its recuperation.

During the next week I felt as though I was living in a thick haze. I continued to take pain medication, which worked as a sedative. My mom, sister and grandmother became my full time nurses. I could not walk or bathe by myself. I found it difficult to eat because of the pain, and a reaction to the potassium supplement I was given. The dosage had been too strong, and it had burned my tongue.

The easiest foods to digest were cooked vegetables and soup. As my appetite returned and the pain decreased, I was able to participate more actively in my recovery process. I was determined to reach a safe weight. I made a decision to eat whatever I craved. When eating seemed like too much of a struggle I would choose something that felt safe, like vegetables or rice. I chose to incorporate french fries and peanut butter for satiety nutrients. Because of my hospital experience my recovery efforts became more focused and progressive. It was crystal clear to me that food and weight were no longer the most important things in my life. My main intention was healing my body and rebuilding my life. I wanted the struggle to be over. I wanted the pain to be over. I wanted the insanity to be over. I knew the only way for that to happen was for me to eat and accept the fact that I had a lot of weight to gain. Since making rules worked for losing weight, I figured it had to work for gaining, too. I decided to eat whenever I became hungry, regardless of the time or where I was. I also decided to eat as much as my body asked for.

When I began realizing the importance of my life and the possibilities I had previously overlooked, eating seemed less torturous. The voices of the eating disorder had been quieted substantially by the threat of death or permanent physical damage. My goal was to make my body as strong and healthy as it had been previously, before the war began. I still had a long way to go, but my decision was made.

The time following my surgery was helpful for physical and emotional healing. I was surrounded by love from Mom, Grandma, Sister, and Kevin. This helped me immensely. I was able to begin understanding my own importance by seeing how important I was to them. I was being re-parented. Also, Kevin would talk with me about my spiritual curiosity and the questions I had. Life seemed to hold more and more possibility for me as I began to reform my thought patterns about self-care.

Physical Changes

During the time I gained most of the weight, I experienced many physical changes. Hot flashes rushed through my body several times per day. My digestive system was irregular. I experienced constant gas. Sometimes I would feel bloated or have stomach cramps. My throat hurt. My head ached. My eyes were sensitive to light. There were times I had to pull off the road because my eyes were tearing from the sunlight. The most troublesome physical repercussion during recovery was fatigue. I took naps daily. I had no energy reserve. My body was working hard to rebuild itself. There was not much fuel left for me to function in life. The smallest activity would drain me, completely. This was frustrating at times. I tried to remember that I was in a healing process, and that my body deserved this time to become strong after all it had been through.

On the psychological and behavioral level, I was not an easy person to deal with. My mood swings were terrible. I was learning how to have emotions again. The main emotion I had not expressed was anger, so I found myself at times filled with rage. Some days I was completely negative and pessimistic. I would yell at people in traffic, and complain constantly. I became territorial with my food. I felt depressed. I didn't fit in anywhere.

Media Messages

It was difficult for me to see advertisements about dieting techniques or to hear people talk about their bodies in a negative way. Sometimes I would mention to someone that I was trying to gain weight, and they would say, "I wish I had that problem." That was hard to hear when I wanted nothing more than to *not* have this problem. I started to feel hopeless about the world. I was trying hard to accept and love myself just as I was, and it seemed as though everywhere I turned there were ads or other media messages telling people they were not good enough just as they were.

Everything seemed to hurt me. When I saw parents yelling at their children or people littering on the street or mistreating their animals I could not hold back from crying or yelling at them. It seemed as though I could not relate to the world. I was lonely and bitter. I barely smiled. I remained reclusive, and wrote in my journals more and more. Dark poetry and angry words poured out of me like a fierce river breaking through a dam. I also began painting. Many of my paintings were dark colors and distorted images expressing my confusion and pain. I was purging all that I had repressed for years. Painting was another way to express my emotions.

I felt trapped in a whirlwind of negativity. This negativity served a purpose. It actually motivated me to recover more quickly. I saw the world as being backwards. My only hope came in thinking that if I became strong and healthy, I would be able to do something to inspire change. It gave me an attitude. With that attitude came confidence.

On the days I felt overwhelmed, I wanted to return to the safe world of my eating disorder. Instead, I would remind myself that my disorder almost killed me. It had stolen my life. I knew that if I went back to it I would not only risk my life, but I would have to do all of the work over again. I was not willing to give any more energy to that monster. It had cost me too much already. I was fighting back. I was beginning to see how the eating disorder had tricked me into underestimating my own worth and strength. I had some valid dreams that deserved to be realized. I was tired of being held back.

When I felt depressed, I let myself feel depressed. I did not ignore the depression; I worked with it. To me, taking medications would only pull a curtain around the depression instead of discovering the reason for it. I spent more time by myself on the days I was sad. I felt quiet and serious. My mom would say, "Where is the old smiling, happy Christine?" Sometimes the old, smiling, happy Christine just wasn't around.

Writing in my journal became my most helpful therapy. It was a productive way of extracting the built up negativity. I was learning a great deal about myself. I was learning why I had an eating disorder. I was beginning to identify the source of my fear. I learned how hard on myself I had been, and what a low opinion of myself I had formed.

Journal writing was also a way to begin using my brain again. The doctors had described how brain centers shut down during long periods of malnutrition. As I nourished my body, I could actually feel my brain awakening. Sometimes my mind moved too fast for my mouth or pen. I struggled with sentences. Sometimes my hand would hurt from writing at a rapid pace. My head would ache from thinking too much. While this process was sometimes uncomfortable, it also had its benefits. My reading comprehension greatly improved. It was exciting to witness the food reversing the effects of my disorder.

Taking The Good With The Bad

A difficult part of re-feeding was learning patience. When I started to feel well again, after reaching a healthy weight, I wanted all of my goals to manifest immediately. I jumped into a new job, joined a band, and went back to school. I often found myself feeling physically overloaded. This resulted in frustration. I wanted to be through with it. Since the weight gain was helping me look normal, I wanted to "be" normal. I was sick of explaining why I could not work full days or stay up late like everyone else my age. I was resenting the same disorder I had previously coveted. Gradually, though, I learned that slowing down my life was only another way to care for myself. I was not used to being kind and loving to myself, and it took a long time to learn.

I slowly began to see that when I did my part, my body would always do the same. I had to be a friend to my body, letting it have the fuel and rest it needed to carry me on in life. I gradually formed a new appreciation for what a wondrous machine the human body is.

As I engaged more in the emotional aspects of my healing, food was less of an issue. I saw that food had been a diversion, keeping me from looking at my own emotional issues. The stronger I felt physically, the more capable I felt of sorting out my tangled emotions. I was peeling away the layers of fear and worry to uncover my true self. I was slowly pulling myself out of the trenches. I was evacuating the battleground. I was taking off the dark comforter of anorexia/bulimia and leaving it behind, among the debris and chaos of war.

A New Me

By the beginning of 1996 I reached a safe weight. I still had some to gain, but I was no longer in danger. I had the stint removed from my ureter, and finally the pain was gone. To celebrate this new phase of my life, I completely changed my appearance. I cut my hair short and dyed it from blonde to auburn. It felt great! When I looked in the mirror I no longer saw the person who had been attacked and weakened by anorexia and bulimia. I saw the new me. I saw the me who was strong enough to take care of myself and gain weight amidst the mental and physical stress of recovery. I believed in life. By that time the weight had stopped bothering me and the voices had become less noticeable. I was having fun with food. I was reading books on proper vegetarian nutrition. I experimented constantly, and gradually learned how to follow a plan of whole grains, beans, vegetables, soy products, nuts, seeds, oils, nut butters, whole grain pastas, breads, and fruits. It was exciting and challenging to be a part of society again. I struggled with media images and my surfacing emotions, but when I was happy, I was happy in a whole new way. The world seemed reachable and fresh.

Treasures Along The Way

During the years of battling anorexia and bulimia something was being born inside of me. It was a whole new person; a person who was dynamic, and vibrant, and ambitious. I was becoming a person who was adamant about making her dreams come true. After making it through such a treacherous war, I felt like I could do anything. In addition to strength I felt a new quality of self-respect. Even though I still had work to do on body image and self-esteem, I finally viewed my life as important. I finally saw my existence as meaningful.

While I was not completely healed emotionally and psychologically, I had collected treasures along the road of struggle which were leading the way. I emerged from the chaos of disorder with a base of power on which I reconstructed my self. Recovery gave me the tools to reach even farther than I could ever have imagined.

Anorexia taught me experientially what I could not have learned any other way. My own self-worth. Through the experience of almost dying, I gained a thirst for living, a hunger for learning, and a passion for growing. This open receptivity to learning led me to the exact situations, teachers, and people I needed in order to continue my inner development.

What Anorexia & Bulimia Mean to Me Now

This brings me to why I am eager to share my story. My eating disorder was simply a step on my stairway of life. It led me to places I would otherwise have missed. It forced me to slow down. This puzzle of an illness pulled me out of the fast paced world. I was forced to look at what I was doing with my time as a human being. I was forced to reclaim my life.

Now I am learning to honor everything that happens to me. I see the value of my successes and my mistakes. There is a rich inner alchemy occurring, even when circumstances seem hopeless. Through every battle, every wound, every struggle, I am coming home to myself.

This is my message to you:

Learn all you can from this strange and amazing process. See it as a chance to regroup and start over. Don't let this unoriginal, template of a disorder become your identity. Don't let it become your life. Scream out loud, "This is it! Today is the day! I have endured enough!"

It is time to nail this experience into its proper place in your life stairway. Climb past it; for all that you overcome leads you closer to attaining your greatest goals. *Decide* on your life - don't just let it *happen* to you. Rescue your true self from the ashes of war! Rise up, and fight for your dreams! Spread your wings, and fly!

CHAPTER FOUR

Food:
From Enemy to Ally

Peace With Food

Anorexia and bulimia turn food into an enemy in order to keep a war going inside of you. Making peace with food means the end of the invader's reign. The key is to convert food from an enemy into an ally.

In a war, the countries in conflict begin developing untrue ideas about one another, and those ideas fuel the fight. Resolution comes on a personal level when both sides see there is no conflict other than the one which has been created to induce war. It is the same with food.

> *"Real healing happens when we dare to breath in the universe, stretching both body and soul to reach for balance and truth. Sometimes, healing moments take forever to arrive. At other times, they fall in our laps with sheer grace, like a feather from an unseen bird."*
>
> *-Kristina Turner*
> **The Self-Healing Cookbook,**
> **Earthtones Press**

The disorder will fight to hold its position of control over you, but your persistence and determination will prove victorious. Make peace with food. Let that peace live within you. Help it grow and blossom, so that it may reach all aspects of your self.

First Things First

The first step is the food. The key is re-feeding. You can deal with the emotional and psychological aspects as you go. A nourished body is stronger and mentally clearer. This clarity makes self-analysis a more attainable goal.

Repairing your relationship with food is the first step in repairing your relationship with your body. It is helpful to notice how food was made into a monster by the invader, when in reality food is a saving grace. As your distorted perception of food is recognized, you will also begin to recognize distorted ideas about your body, and your self as a whole.

Food is the substance of life. It allows your body to continue functioning; and without your body, you could not be here. The invader has been convincing you that you are different, and do not need food to survive. It has transferred your stifled negative emotions onto food, creating fear and hatred. It takes time and effort to replace these unhealthy ideas about food, but this is all part of exposing the eating disorder, and reclaiming your power.

Recovery begins by simply changing your behavior. The only way to change a toxic activity is to replace it with a healthy one. Think of it as a garden, no matter how many weeds you pull, there will always be more weeds. The real power of the garden is in feeding and caring for the healthy plants. A certain amount of weeding will be required, but if you spend most of your time strengthening the healthy plants, soon they will fill up the garden, leaving little room for weeds to grow.

Eating disorders can inspire some of these thoughts:

- I have more energy when I don't eat.
- Eating makes me feel sick.
- Eating is a sign of weakness.
- Skinny is pretty.
- The only time I am happy is when I am losing weight.

All of these statements are fuel for the illness. They are generated by the invader as a control mechanism.

Food cannot be malicious. It cannot *want* to make you overweight. The invader gives food an imaginary evil personality. It tells you food is an enemy who wants to make you fat. *Food has no intentions*. It simply plays its role; nourishing the body. All other meanings for food are created by the disorder. By keeping food an enemy, the eating disorder maintains control. It separates you from the truth. It divides and conquers.

It is helpful to confront distorted perceptions of food, and identify the originator of these perceptions as anorexia/bulimia. Doing this creates a united front which can hold strong against the invader. We can access the rational mind by looking closely at whether our perceptions are fact or fiction.

JOURNAL BREAK: Redefining Food

- What does food mean to you?

- What role does food play in your life?

- What emotions surface when you think about food?

- Is your description of food based on ideas from the invader, or from the part of you who wants to be well? If your description came from the eating disorder, try writing another description. Try describing some positive things about food.

- What lies does the invader tell you about food?

Food As Medicine

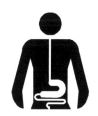 All living things need food for survival, including your body. Your body is an energy transformer. It takes the energy of food and turns it into energy for our thoughts, emotions, ideas, and activities. The body performs these miracles on its own, without our being aware of it. We need to step back and let it do its job. The body and food have a naturally harmonious relationship. The invader's goal is to disrupt this balance. In order to heal your damaged relationship with food, and heal the body, food must become medicine.

Anorexia and bulimia are illnesses, and food is part of the cure. Food nourishes the body, repairs lost tissues and bone density, re-ignites brain function and reproductive function, gives energy for thoughts and feelings, and keeps you warm. Even malnourished animals instinctively eat more to become healthier.

 A young woman in the support group once used her dog as an example of food working as medicine. The dog had been ill, lost weight, and displayed low energy. Each day the dog would only stand up and walk when she needed to eat, and then she would rest. The dog ate twice as much as usual, because her instincts knew food would help her become strong again. When the dog became healthy again, her appetite returned to normal. Animals function on instinct. That instinct exists in human beings, but can be covered up by contorted thoughts and feelings related to eating disorders.

Redefining Healthy Eating

Eating disorders can begin with a desire to eat in a healthier way. This is a positive intention which can help to improve quality of life. The problem begins when the invader takes control of forming your definition of healthy eating. While under the invader's control, you lose touch with rational ideas of what is beneficial for the body. In fact, food no longer has anything to do with health and well-being. Within an eating disorder, food becomes only something to control. As the invader's reign continues, more foods become forbidden. This is not because the foods suddenly become "bad." It is to pull you further into the secluded delusion of the invader's world. If it can gain more power by doing so, the invader will convince you that *water* is too fattening to drink. The invader is not concerned with your survival, it is only concerned with *its* survival. It will use whatever conniving methods it can to devour you. You must stop fueling the invader's perception of food, and build your own.

"I Can Relate To That!"
Redefining Healthy Eating

During my healing process I was able to transform my view of food. My disorder had convinced me that food was something to be feared, an enemy to be avoided. I eventually learned that food had been falsely accused. I came to honor food for all of the delightful nourishment it provides. I recognize it as fuel for the body.

I enjoy cooking. In fact, cooking is one way I generate income. I eat a balanced vegetarian diet which includes organic vegetables, grains, oils, soy products, nuts and seeds, all-natural desserts, and some fruit. I have repaired my relationship with my body, and I listen to its signs of hunger and fullness. What was once my greatest symbol of anxiety and sadness is now a source of joy and fulfillment.

In 1996 I began seeking alternative forms of medicine to treat endometriosis and a weak kidney. I was tired of being in pain, for it affected my ability to work consistently, and decreased my energy level. I consulted both a chiropractor and an herbalist, which provided some relief. Then in 1997, I met an acupuncturist/macrobiotic counselor named Stefan Brink - and everything changed.

He spent 3 1/2 hours with me during my first appointment. I filled out extensive patient history forms filled with strange questions I had never seen before. Everything was extremely thorough. I told him about every symptom I had, right down to my achy knees and cold hands and feet. I was amazed when he explained that according to Chinese medicine every symptom was related. I felt incredibly relieved! He was able to trace all of my ailments back to two main sources. He told me to stop taking all herbs and vitamins, and explained that it is best receive all nutrients from food alone. This made sense to me. He began teaching me about Chinese dietary theory which has been healing people for thousands of years. This felt much more credible than modern medicine, which was only a few hundred years old, and treated the symptoms rather than the root causes of illness.

He gave me some new ideas of what to incorporate into my diet to begin feeling better, and gave me a few natural foods cookbooks based on the Chinese dietary system. He showed me foods I had never heard of, including varieties of sea vegetables, which could provide many trace minerals and B vitamins - nutrients in which the body can become deficient while eating vegetarian.

At the end of my first appointment he asked me if I wanted to get better, and I said, "More than anything."

His confident response was, "Then together we will heal you."

When I left his office, I was a new person. I was immersed in a new found hope that I would not have to be in pain for the rest of my life. Many other doctors had made me think I was only imagining my ailments. He was sure I would make progress.

I immediately began studying and experimenting in order to become familiar with the ingredients in macrobiotic cooking. Within one month of receiving regular treatments and cooking in this more natural way, I was free of pain and had more energy than ever before.

My only wish is that I had learned about the healing properties of food at the beginning of my recovery. I could have chosen to prepare foods that were gently nourishing and building for the body. This would have made recovery a little easier, which is why I felt compelled to share this information with those embarking upon a similar journey of healing. We need to view food as medicine during recovery, so why not choose the highest quality and most appropriate medicine?

ACTIVITY BREAK: Write a new definition of healthy eating

Do some research about nutrition. Consult several resources about health. Take a nutrition course at a community college. Check out some books at the health food store. Read some natural health magazines. Talk to a doctor. Talk to a chef. Ask your family members and friends how they would define healthy eating. Take notes on what you learn, then review the material you have collected.

Now write your own definition of healthy eating. How would you like to feel? Energized? Alive? Alert? What food combinations could help your body feel that way? What foods, and how much food, does the body need to maintain its normal processes?

This exercise will begin to challenge the invader's distorted ideas about food with scientific fact, and common sense.

Making The Decision

Winning this war against the invader depends on the solidity of your decision. Your decision to carry through with re-feeding is an important promise to your self; perhaps the most important promise you will ever make. Keeping this promise will prove to be the most powerful way to raise your self-esteem. Remind yourself every day that you have made the decision to re-feed. Declare it out loud every morning when you awake. Let the strength of your conviction carry you through the rough days. Do it because you said you would. Use the insights, ideas, and activities offered in this book. Perfection is not necessary, but continuous effort is.

In the dark world of an eating disorder, controlling food is confining and damaging. A greater sense of control and satisfaction will be yours as you heal the body and learn self-care. It is deeper than the illusionary control found in an eating disorder. By letting go of monsters, we make room for angels.

Journal Break: Finding Your "Why"
(After finishing this journal exercise, keep it close by. Read it often. It will remind you why you are taking on this difficult fight. It will bring you courage during challenging moments.)

- Why do you want to recover? What are some things you are going to do once you are healthy? What dreams and goals are on hold due to your disorder?

- Write a pro/con list about your eating disorder. On one side of the space below, list all of the things you like about having anorexia and/or bulimia. What does it do for you? Why are you reluctant to let it go? On the other side of the space below, list all of the negative aspects of the eating disorder. What are you ready to let go of? How has the disorder affected you physically, emotionally, and mentally? How has it affected your relationships? What has the eating disorder taken away from your life?

<u>PRO</u>   <u>CON</u>

ACTIVITY BREAK: Affirm your decision!

Find some construction paper, cardboard, or posterboard. Choose paint, crayons, markers, or colored pencils with which you would enjoy working. Select a mission statement for your recovery. Think of it as your battle cry, your mantra, your slogan. Use the ideas listed below, or think of some yourself. After selecting your phrase, use the art materials to create a sign or poster to display the words. Make them fancy. Sprinkle them with glitter, or glue some pieces of fabric on them. Make as many signs as you would like. Tape one to the wall next to your bed and say it to yourself as soon as you awaken each morning. Hang them in places around your house where you will see them often. When you pass them during the day, say the slogans out loud. Make it fun! Say them in different accents, sing them, scream them!

- I HAVE DECIDED TO HEAL!
- I CAN DO IT!
- I WANT TO LIVE!
- I WILL RECOVER!
- I RECLAIM MY LIFE!
- NO INVADER ALLOWED!

Affirming your decision to recover by creating these motivational posters, and using them often, will provide some of the fuel needed by the part of you who wants to live. Remember, you have to do something different to achieve different results in your life. These mission statements can begin the process of forming new neural pathways in the brain which support the healing process.

Remember, food is not your enemy. Food is your medicine. Food is your friend. Food is your ally. You have the power to decide what food means to you, and what role it will play in your life. You are embarking upon a challenging and rewarding journey. Accepting help from food will make the benefits of healing surface more quickly.

<u>SELF-CHECK</u>

Shade in how much of you is still controlled by the eating disorder.

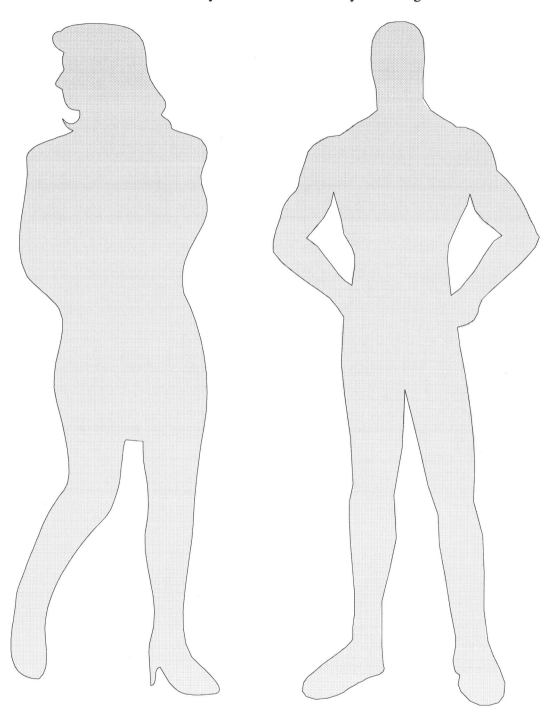

CHAPTER FIVE

 Gentle Nutrition

A Helping Hand

This chapter offers a different perspective. Use it as an option, along with other recovery tools. It is wise to use all resources available to increase awareness and promote recovery. Check with a nutritionist and a doctor to be sure all necessary nutrients are being taken in. Perhaps the best way to utilize the suggestions in this section is to use them in conjunction with a food plan from a nutritionist.

This section describes a grain based nutritional program of three meals and two snacks per day, in which all food is eaten in its most natural form. It incorporates grains, vegetables, soups, sea vegetables, fruits, beans, soy products, nuts, seeds, and oils. Many natural food cookbooks also include fish and other forms of animal protein in moderation. This section will focus on the vegetarian foods.

Non-animal foods are much less intimidating for a recovering anorexic or bulimic. Recovering with a vegetarian program is possible if the necessary nutritional research is done. This can be achieved through cookbooks, health magazines, and by talking to people knowledgeable in alternative healing arts.

A vegetarian nutritional program is not suitable for every person recovering from an eating disorder. Using vegetarianism as an excuse not to incorporate fats into the diet, or to subtly continue with eating disorder behavior, is not the purpose of this section. If this issue becomes a conflict between parents and their children, a compromise can be reached. Try eating whole grains, vegetables, fruits, nuts, and soy protein, and incorporating healthy animal products like organic dairy, eggs, farm-raised fish, and organic meats, if desired. If you truly want to heal using a vegetarian program, it is possible; but you must be armed with knowledge.

Part of the fear involved in recovery comes from the manner in which some hospital programs direct re-feeding. Many of the meals are foods greatly feared by those suffering, and are difficult for the body to digest, especially after restricting.

If your house had been damaged by harsh weather, would you not want to go about the repairs in the most well-planned, productive fashion? You would want to hire the right company, and use the highest quality, most sturdy building supplies.

Your body is your house during this lifetime. If time and effort are taken to help it heal sensibly, it will become strong and healthy. It will offer enough energy and alertness for you to reach your every dream. It makes sense to ease into eating again so that your body, mind, and spirit all have time to adjust.

Learning how to prepare and eat food in a more natural way gradually creates a new lifestyle, filled with healthy living, balance, and confidence. The balance reached in the food helps bring balance internally, as well. Many people with eating disorders who are vegetarian or vegan have a belief in animal rights, as well as environmental concerns which are completely valid. This program offers a healthy recovery option which respects these beliefs. While providing all necessary nutrients, gently re-introducing food will not scare a person back into the disorder.

A New Re-feeding Program

According to The Self-Healing Cookbook, by Kristina Turner, Earthtones Press, there are three basic principles to guide you toward a whole foods diet that restores your body's natural, self-healing abilities:

1. Eat in harmony with nature.
2. Balance nature's forces in cooking.
3. Use food to create desired effects.

 "Eat in harmony with nature" means eating traditional, whole, unrefined foods, locally grown, when possible, and cooked appropriately for each season. It is important to choose foods which are organically grown and produced, which means they are free of pesticides and herbicides. Organic foods are easier on the healing body. When eating organically, the body does not have to put energy into discarding the chemicals, and can use its energy for digesting and absorbing nutrients, which are more abundant in organic foods.

Eating less-refined foods is important while re-feeding as well. This means incorporating whole grains like brown rice, millet, and quinoa, instead of eating low quality refined grains, such as bagels or cold cereal. Unrefined foods offer a more lasting energy source, and help to balance blood sugar.

Becoming familiar with foods which are most nutritionally beneficial in each season can also aid in recovery. For example, sweet vegetables are harvested in the late summer/early autumn, so it is most beneficial to highlight squash, parsnips, carrots, onions, and other sweet vegetables at this time. Sweet vegetables, sweet brown rice, and millet naturally nourish the stomach, spleen and pancreas. These organs are all intensely out of balance during the beginning stages of re-feeding. It is helpful to incorporate these foods into your recovery program. It is possible to form a symbiotic relationship with the earth's natural cycles, and to give your body foods which will help it along the re-feeding path.

"Balance natural forces in cooking" means seeking a healthful blend of warm and cool, heavy and light, crunchy and mushy, salty and sweet, easy and difficult, basic and creative. Meals can be prepared in an attempt to balance the two forces of the universe, yin and yang. Yin is expansive, cold, and sweet; yang is contractive, hot, and salty. It is most beneficial to base meals around foods found in the middle of the spectrum, such as whole grains, vegetables, beans, sea vegetables, local fruits, and nuts. Eating large amounts of raw, spicy, or cold foods may cause trouble with digestion. Less extreme, cooked foods are easier on the body. This gentle idea of balancing works as an assistant to the body during its healing process, without it exhausted.

"Use food to create desired effects" means cooking and eating for balance. Food choices affect your body, mood, and energy level. These treasures of knowledge in relation to healing the body offer many benefits, which do not end with recovery. This information can allow one to become healthy and stay healthy. Learn how to treat many common ailments with food. Discover what foods to eat the day before a final exam to help with focus and concentration. Know what foods and cooking methods are warming in the winter (or during recovery), and cooling in the summer.

Through reading, experimenting, and speaking with someone knowledgeable in natural foods cooking, it is possible to formulate a re-feeding plan which is gradual, nourishing, and gentle.

Becoming Familiar With Natural Foods

Many people are unfamiliar with the ingredients in natural food cookbooks, and feel lost in a health food store. This section defines foods which are commonly used in the books recommended at the end of this chapter, as well as in the recipes listed in the next section.

Whole Grains

Amaranth: The tiniest of grains, amaranth cooks into a delicious, nourishing breakfast cereal. It is soothing, smooth, and alkalizing to the system.

Brown Rice: Brown rice is unpolished and comes complete with bran and germ. Most rice eaten in America is white and stripped of nutrients and fiber. The taste of brown rice is slightly richer than white. Making the transition is worth the many health benefits. There are many varieties of brown rice available. *Short Grain Brown Rice* is small and oval shaped. It is best to use in temperate or cool climates. *Medium Grain Brown Rice* is slightly longer than short grain and is a wonderful variety to use year round. *Long Grain Brown Rice* is light and fluffy. It is close to white rice in texture, so it might be the best choice for those making the switch. *Sweet Brown Rice* is a wonderful choice during re-feeding. Its sweet flavor makes it nourishing for the stomach, spleen, and pancreas; all organs heavily affected by eating disorders. It is sticky, soft, and easily digestible.

Millet: Millet is small, round, and golden. It becomes fluffy when cooked, and with extra water added during cooking, it can be turned into porridge. Millet is alkalizing to the blood. It is also a grain which nourishes the middle burner (stomach, spleen, pancreas) which makes it a gentle choice for those re-feeding.

Barley: With a texture firmer than brown rice, barley adds variety to a whole grain program. Barley can be added to soups to thicken them and add nutritional value. Barley can also be eaten as a morning cereal.

Buckwheat: Also known as kasha. This hearty grain is tastier when roasted before cooking. It cooks fast and has an earthy flavor. Can be made into grain burgers, eaten as a side dish, or enjoyed for breakfast with dried fruit.

Quinoa: Quinoa is a strong grain, high in protein. Its seeds were found in a pyramid in Egypt. When they were planted, surprisingly they grew. Quinoa was termed the "super-grain" because of its strength. It is light, fluffy, and cute.

Wheat: Most often, wheat is ground into flour for bread and noodles, offering a more beneficial variety of these favorites. Whole wheat berries can be cooked and eaten as a breakfast cereal.

Proteins

Beans: A wonderful source of iron, vitamins, protein, and fiber, beans are a must in any vegetarian food plan. Varieties include:
- aduki beans - red and strengthening
- black turtle beans - great for soups and burritos
- black soy beans - slightly crunchy and healing. Drinking the juice left after cooking helps heal and balance the female reproductive system
- chickpeas - gentle and nourishing in hummus, or soups
- kidney beans - wonderful fall bean
- lentils - quick-cooking, yummy in soups
- mung beans - small and tasty
- navy beans - white, winter bean
- pinto beans - perfect to mash up for "re-fried" taste
- yellow or green split peas- melt as they cook- delicious soups

Seitan: Sometimes called "wheat meat". Made from whole wheat gluten. Very high in protein, popular meat substitute. Can be made from scratch, or purchased frozen or refrigerated in health food stores.

Tofu: Soy bean curd, high in protein and calcium. When fresh, it looks like a white block of feta cheese stored in water. Stays fresh in the refrigerator up to one week, if water is changed daily. It soaks up the flavors with which it is cooked. Many health food stores offer varieties which are already baked with spices, and ready to eat or add to salads, soups and grains. Silken tofu in a box can be used to make non-dairy, high protein puddings, "cream" pies, or sauces.

Tempeh: A cultured soybean product with a nutty texture. Comes frozen or refrigerated in cakes. Can be baked, broiled, stir-fried, steamed, braised, or marinated. High in protein, iron, and vitamin B-12, which is unusual for non-animal proteins.

Tahini: Sesame seed butter originally from the Middle East. Wonderful satiety nutrient high in protein. Easy to use in sauces, soups, desserts, and hummus.

Nuts and Nut Butters: Now available in many varieties: cashew, almond, filbert, peanut, macadamia, pecan, walnut, sunflower. Tasty, high in protein, and versatile. A wonderful place to start incorporating lipids into the re-feeding program. Eat nuts by themselves or with raisins, on yogurt, or with fresh fruit. Eat nut butters on toast, with an apple, or alone.

Vegetables. Fruits, and Sea Vegetables

Vegetables:
- greens: collards, kale, mustard greens, broccoli, dandelions, spinach, and watercress.
- lettuces: Bibb, Boston, chicory, escarole, curly, romaine, red and green leaf.
- cabbages: bok choy, Chinese cabbage, savoy, red cabbage, white cabbage, and nappa.
- sweet roots: onions, sweet potatoes, beets, parsnips, yams, and carrots.
- other roots: ginger, garlic, lotus root, burdock root, daikon, radish, turnip, burdock, rutabaga.
- autumn treats: Butternut, buttercup, scan squash, corn, and pumpkins.
- others: cauliflower, brussel sprouts, green and yellow beans, avocado, tomato, snow peas,
- scallions, red and green peppers, zucchini, yellow squash, mushrooms, parsley, potatoes.

Fruits: During recovery, I suggest cooking or baking fruit. This makes it easier to digest and more soothing to the body. Raw foods are hard on the stomach, and have a cooling effect on the body. The most gentle fruits are apples, pears, peaches, plums, and blackberries.

Sea Vegetables: A wonderful source of vitamins and minerals. These foods are not widely known, although they are extremely healing, and rich in nutrients. Arame is the most mild tasting sea vegetable. Dulse and kelp are salty and are available granulated to sprinkle on food. Kombu can be cooked with beans to tenderize them, and help reduce gas. Hijiki is the strongest tasting sea vegetable, and helps the body strengthen. Wakame is a nice addition to soups. Agar-agar is a natural gelatin used to make vegan "jello" (kanten). Nori can be used to make vegan sushi rolls. Try to keep an open mind with these new textures and appearances. I recommend at least a small portion of sea vegetable each day in a vegan or vegetarian nutritional program, because of the trace mineral and B-12 content.

Other Whole Foods

Miso: Miso is an important food during re-feeding. Miso is a salty paste made out of soybeans and whole grains. The beans and grains are cooked and aged with salt in wooden tubs for two months to several years. Miso is rich in enzymes to help with digestion. It contains friendly bacteria to help maintain a healthy intestinal flora. Miso contains every amino acid required to build a complete protein. It is one of the most healing foods in existence. It can be used to flavor soups, sauces, mashed potatoes, or casseroles. Darker miso is usually more medicinal and used in colder months of the year. I suggest unpasturized miso, which is sold in the refrigerated section of the health food store. It is important to keep miso below the boiling point to keep the enzymes alive.

Umeboshi: A pickled plum. Available whole, as a paste, or in a liquid concentrate. It is sour and salty in flavor. Umeboshi is highly alkaline and boosts energy, bolsters the immune system, and treats nausea. Umeboshi vinegar can be used in spring and summer salad dressings.

Kuzu: Kuzu is a white and chunky root which looks a lot like chalk. It is used as a thickener for soups, sauces, gravies, and desserts. Kuzu is a gentle, alkalinizing, soothing food with many medicinal qualities.

Sea Salt: It is important to switch to sea salt from commercial table salt, especially for re-feeding. Commercial salt is refined and mixed with sugar and sodium bicarbonate to retain its whiteness. It puts stress on vital organs, and decreases energy in the body. Sea salt is thicker, coarser, and more moist than commercial salt, as well as richer in taste. Sea salt aids in digestion, and offers a natural, mineral balance. High quality sea salt has a texture similar to wet sand.

Oils: Unrefined oils are the most healthy. Sesame, olive, and safflower oils are wonderful for sautéing and for use in salad dressings. Corn oil is great for baking. Oils lubricate the digestive system, and give more energy than carbohydrates!

Pickles: Pickled cucumbers, beets, green beans, and cabbage are all extremely helpful with digestion. I recommend eating something pickled with every meal.

Keifer and yogurt: Keifer is a cultured dairy product similar to yogurt. It is thinner, and can be used in cereal or eaten plain. It is available in health food stores in plain or fruit flavors, or you can make your own (see recipe in The Body Ecology Diet, which is cited in the Book Suggestion List at the end of the book). Keifer and yogurt are rich in calcium and acidophilus. Acidophilus is friendly bacteria in the digestive tract. Without it digestion can be difficult. Keifer can aid in healing and restructuring the intestines after abuse from eating disorder behavior. I highly recommend it if you can tolerate dairy products.

The Truth About Fat

Fats found in oils, nuts, seeds, nut butters, some vegetables, and other foods, are just as beneficial to our bodies as all the other foods on earth. There is room for everything in a healthy nutritional program. The labeling of foods as 'good' or 'bad' creates an internal police squad that follows a person around enforcing restrictions.

Almost every person with an eating disorder fears and detests any food containing fat. This relationship must be repaired for a successful recovery. Below is a list of all the positive things lipids provide for the body. Try to read this information with the logical mind rather than the invader mind.

- regulates: blood pressure, blood clotting, hormone levels, stomach secretions, contraction of muscles, and body temperature.
- keeps skin soft and smooth.
- helps hair stay thick and shiny.
- found in the membrane of every single cell of the body; human cells cannot exist without fat.
- serves as a shock absorber for every joint.
- protects and supports organs.
- assists in the stabilization of mood.
- helps alleviate depression.
- great giver of energy.
- promotes restful sleep.
- lubricates the digestive system and eases constipation.
- pads every nerve cell, allowing nerves to continue functioning.
- keeps the body warm.

"I Can Relate To That!"
Fear of Fat

I remember beginning the re-feeding process without incorporating fats into my nutritional program. I procrastinated adding them because I thought they would make me gain excessive amounts of weight immediately. My moods remained unstable. My depression did not lift. I did not have any energy. My eating disorder was still taking up quite a bit of space in my brain, and it was convincing me that I could recover without eating any fats, and without gaining weight. This was the most difficult lie to stop believing.

I had been sure that fat would make me overweight. I was terrified of it. I would cry sometimes just thinking about eating foods with fat. It took a long time for me to learn that these satiety nutrients are not only beneficial to human health, they are absolutely necessary.

When I was told I would have to be hospitalized if I did not stop losing weight, I started adding fat with a teaspoon of peanut butter every day. It was frightening, but I gradually became used to the taste and eventually saw that the peanut butter was not making me gain weight any faster. With this realization, I actually began looking forward to my peanut butter treat each day, and was able to increase it each week. When I started to feel better because of it, I overcame my fear even faster. When I had been eating peanut butter regularly for about one month, I actually felt more alive. I had more energy, I slept better, the negative thoughts were weakening, and my depression even began to lift. I was happier in general. Later in my recovery, I stopped thinking about fat altogether, and worked my way up to the recommended amount per day. The results were astounding, and I was able to keep myself out of the hospital.

Here are some ideas for how to gradually add fat to your diet:

Nutty Nutrition: Purchase a bag or jar of your favorite nut. Every day with your lunch eat one nut. Just one nut. This is a completely safe and gentle beginning. After a week, increase to one nut with lunch and one with dinner. After that week, increase to one nut with breakfast, one with lunch, and one with dinner. Now you are used to the taste and texture, and should be able to see that the nuts are not making you gain weight any faster. In the fourth week, increase to two nuts with each meal. In the fifth, four nuts with each meal. By the sixth week it will be obvious that the nuts are not making you overweight, and the fear will begin to subside.

> **Quick Tip:** Almonds are the easiest nut to digest.

Satiety sauté: Every other day for dinner, sauté some vegetables in oil and water for a side dish. Choose an oil with which you are most comfortable. Choose a vegetable like carrots, onion, broccoli, zucchini, or yellow squash. Place one teaspoon of oil and one teaspoon of water in a pan on the stove. Heat the mixture until liquidy, and add vegetables. Sauté for 3-5 minutes, stirring.

Teaspoon 0' Nut Butter Try spreading a teaspoon of peanut, cashew, almond, or soy butter on a piece of toast every other day. As you become more used to it, incorporate it daily. Add jelly for variety. If you don't like toast, warm up the nut butter, and use it as a fresh fruit dip.

> **Helpful Hint:** If the word "fat" is difficult for you to use, here are some easy substitutes:
> - Lipids
> - Cell Liners
> - Satiety Nutrients
> - Energies

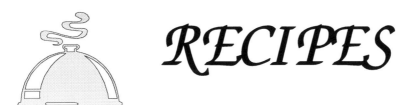

RECIPES

Here are some gentle, simple recipes, which may help ignite the re-feeding process. I have included variations and additions with most recipes. Incorporate these as you feel ready. Remember to be patient with yourself, yet firm enough to make progress in your recovery.

Creamy Amaranth

Amaranth is a whole grain with a mildly sweet taste. Whole and uncooked, the grains are tiny and round. When cooked, they gel together, creating a creamy hot cereal. Amaranth is alkalizing to the blood. Amaranth is available in most health food stores. In the summer, try amaranth flakes with cold milk, soymilk, or ricemilk.

½ cup amaranth
1½ cups cold water

Combine amaranth and water in a medium saucepan. Bring to a boil. Reduce heat and simmer for 20-25 minutes, stirring occasionally. Serve by itself or with milk, soymilk, or ricemilk.

Variations:
- Add two tablespoons of raisins and a dash of cinnamon.
- Add one tablespoon of chopped walnuts before serving.
- Add fresh chopped apples, pears, or banana during the last 10 minutes of cooking.
- Add one tablespoon of any nut butter before serving (cashew, almond, peanut, soy, filbert).

Sweet Rice

This short grain brown rice is a soothing, sweet tasting grain, rich in vitamins and minerals. It is a perfect late Summer/early Autumn food, and nourishes the stomach, spleen, and pancreas. When cooked, sweet rice becomes soft and sticky. This grain is easy to digest, and wonderful for re-feeding.

½ cup sweet brown rice
1 cup water

Combine water and rice in a medium saucepan. Bring to a boil, cover, and reduce temperature to low. Simmer for about 30 minutes until rice is soft and sticky. Serve with steamed kale or baked squash. Enjoy as a breakfast cereal with milk, soymilk, or keifer and raisins.

Baked Squash

Use buttercup, butternut, or acorn squash. Squash is soothing and warming to the stomach, spleen, and pancreas. It will help keep blood sugar balanced, which is important during re-feeding.

Cut squash in half and place face down in a baking dish. Pour in about ½ inch of water and bake for 35-45 minutes. Squash is done when fork can easily pierce the skin. Sprinkle baked squash with sea salt and cinnamon.

Variations:
- Scoop squash out of its shell and mix with toasted walnuts and currants.
- Add a touch of brown rice syrup or honey to sweeten for squash pudding.
- Puree squash in a blender with 1 cup water and 3 tablespoons dissolved mellow or chick pea miso for creamy squash soup.

Sweet Corn and Arame

Arame is mild tasting and extremely high in minerals. It is also a vegan source of B-12. Corn is a sweet vegetable, so it will be soothing to the digestive system as long as it is chewed well. Try cutting the corn fresh off the cob. Ginger adds zip to the dish, and makes it more warming. Ginger is also a good remedy for nausea. Ginger can be added to any dish during recovery.

½ ounce arame
½ cup corn, cut off cob
3 tablespoons fresh grated ginger

Soak arame for 10 minutes in enough water to cover it. Place in a medium saucepan and heat at medium. Let simmer for 10 minutes and add some tamari or shoyu. Add corn and simmer for 3 minutes more. Grate ginger and squeeze juice into pot. Drain and serve warm.

Rice Cream

Short grain, medium grain, or sweet rice can be used to make rice cream. Rice cream is one of the most gentle foods, so it is perfect for the beginning stages of re-feeding.

½ cup brown rice
1½ cups water

Combine rice and water in sauce pan. Bring to boil, reduce heat and simmer for 45-50 minutes. For creamier rice, use more water and cook longer.

Variations:
- Add cinnamon, maple syrup, and toasted walnuts for a breakfast treat.
- Use ½ cup soymilk in place of ½ cup of water.
- Add a few tablespoons of granola.

 Apple-Kuzu Drink
I suggest organic apple juice for this warm treat. This is a soothing, slightly thick beverage, perfect for a cold winter evening.

1½ cups apple juice
pinch of sea salt
1 tablespoon kuzu root

Warm apple juice and sea salt over medium heat until simmering. Dissolve kuzu in two tablespoons of cold water and stir into apple juice. Let simmer until drink is slightly thick. Serve warm with a cinnamon stick.

Variations:
* Use as a sauce over frozen yogurt, soy ice cream, rice ice cream, fruit flavored keifer, or dairy ice cream.

Creating A Fresh Perspective

While preparing food remind yourself that you are in a healing process and this food is medicine. The ingredients are gifts from Mother Earth. Try to see cooking and eating from a brand new perspective. You are participating in an activity humans have been doing for millions of years.

Food is sacred. Meals have been the center of celebrations, ceremonies, and life-changing events for generations.

Preparing food holds a great source of energy for you. It simply depends on how you choose to see it. Try to make contact with a new part of yourself; the part of yourself which has been bound and gagged by your disorder. Let that part of you prepare the meal. Let that part of you enjoy the scents and textures of what you are preparing. Remember that you are more than your disorder.

Before eating, it may be a good idea to say a few words, expressing your gratitude. Here are some ideas of what you could say:

* I am grateful for this second chance at life.
* I am thankful for this healing food.
* I acknowledge this food as the substance which gives me life.
* I am grateful for this medicine from Mother Earth.
* I welcome the possibility of being healed by this food.

Or, choose a phrase from a book which expresses a fresh perspective on food, like this quote from Kahlil Gibran's The Prophet:

"When you crush an apple with your teeth, say to it in your heart,
'Your seeds shall live in my body, and the buds of your tomorrow
shall blossom in my heart, and your fragrance shall be my breath,
and together we shall rejoice through all the seasons.'"

Food can be viewed as a symbol of the future. It is the train carrying you across the barren lands of battle into the lush, lively fields of freedom. When food appeared as an enemy, it was a distorted perception, forced on you by the eating disorder. It was all part of its control over you. Making the decision to transform your ideas about food is a large part of reclaiming control over your life.

FOOD IS SACRED, AND SO ARE YOU!

CHAPTER SIX

What to Expect During Re-feeding

Out of the Fog

Every person's body is unique. Therefore, every person's physical, psychological, and emotional reactions to re-feeding will differ. The length of the process depends on the length of time eating-disorder behavior was practiced, specific ways of restricting or purging, and consistency with recovery. This section will describe some common reactions to re-feeding.

> *"The miracle, or the power, that elevates the few is to be found in their industry, application, and perseverance under the prompting of a brave, determined spirit.*
> *-Mark Twain*

The process of re-nourishing the body will be difficult. It requires determination, consistency, diligence, and courage. This effort will pay off in numerous ways. It is like stepping out of a thick fog into the sunshine. Discoveries will be made. Strengths will be revealed. Knowledge will be attained. We are all students of life, and this is a potent lesson.

The first part of re-feeding is the most challenging. It means taking a giant step into unfamiliar territory. It is uncomfortable at first. However, as the body is brought into balance, the unfamiliar becomes the familiar. The sunshine begins to feel good after a while, and the idea of going back into the fog loses its charm.

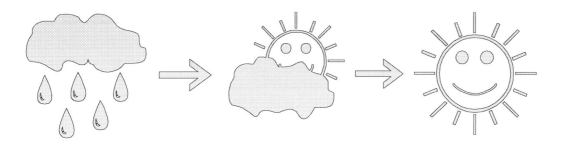

Overcoming the Fear of Food

Undoubtedly, fear will be the first obstacle to overcome. The part of your mind still connected with the eating disorder will attack the part which is trying to heal. Old, familiar, toxic thoughts will flood in, trying to control your behavior.

They may be thoughts like:

•I can't eat all of this food.

•I'm going to die if I eat this.

•Eating this food reverses all the hard work I put into losing weight.

•If I start eating, I won't be able to stop.

•If I start gaining weight everyone will look at me strangely, and think I am out of control.

These are toxic thoughts, which do not represent who you truly are. You are more than an eating disorder. You have a choice. Food is not your enemy; it is your medicine. Remember your motivation. Become a warrior fighting for your life!

Fear will manifest itself into physical symptoms. Usually the first week is the hardest and most filled with uncomfortable reactions to eating. It may be less frightening if you have some idea of what to expect. The body needs patience and love. It has tried to please you by becoming used to not eating. It is going to take time for it to switch gears and become used to digestion. Take your time. Be your body's partner.

Here are some ways fear may affect the body:

- creating the illusion that the esophagus is filled up to the back of the mouth
- creating the illusion that the throat is swollen or that swallowing is impossible
- nausea
- stomach cramps
- bloating
- gas pains
- food is stuck in the stomach and won't move

It makes sense that your stomach may bloat, and your intestines may produce gas. These organs have not been used properly, and have to re-learn their instinctive functions. Digestion is slowed down as well, because the stomach is re-learning how to use and regulate its acids. While these reactions are uncomfortable, they do go away with time. The more consistent the food intake, the faster these symptoms subside.

Try to remain calm and relaxed. Talk or write about what you are feeling in your body. If you do not express this experience, it can build up more fear and create more difficulty. When you talk out loud about this process, it becomes more manageable. Part of the eating disorder's trick is to make you think it is not okay to talk about it. This is another way it maintains control.

JOURNAL BREAK: What Is Fear?

•What does fear feel like to you?

•Is the feeling of fear associated with any colors or images?

•Can you find or draw a picture of your fear?

Preparing for Battle

When food is near, the invader will attack; firing torturing negative self-talk into the mind, creating much stress and panic for the person recovering. This section offers an arsenal for a counter-attack.

> *"Everything is happening for the best. Go bravely through the dark night of the soul."*
> -*Swami Paramatmananda Puri*
> <u>*On the Road to Freedom*</u>

Burning the Lies

Place a candle, a heavy-bottomed pot, some slips of paper, and a pencil on the table during your meals. When the invader attacks with negative self-talk, write out whatever it tells you on a piece of paper. Light it with the candle, and let it burn in the pot. Do this throughout the meal, as often as necessary. This activity can be a powerful way to burn away toxic thoughts, in order to make room for loving thoughts. Eventually, you may want to try writing a replacement thought for every thought burned. For example, if the invader says, "You are going to get fat if you eat that," you could burn that thought, and replace it with, "This food is saving my life."

Planning, Preparation and Shopping

It can be helpful for the whole family to plan and prepare meals together. If you live alone, you may want to ask a close friend or sibling to share the process. If you discuss negative thoughts immediately, the eating disorder automatically loses power. Give more of an effort to making the entire process safe and fun. It may be helpful to choose meals from a cookbook which feels safe (see Book Suggestion List at the end of this chapter), or from the recipes in chapter five.

Choose a meal, and then go to a store to purchase the ingredients. Some people feel more comfortable in a small corner health food store. Others prefer fancy international markets. Shop where it feels safest. If shopping is too difficult at first, make the list with a friend or loved one, and ask that person to make the trip for you.

Challenges to new horizons are necessary, but part of self-love is accepting the gradual nature of recovery, and learning to use patience.

Breathing

Breathing is an activity which will help in all areas of recovery, especially re-feeding. Most people take shallow breaths, into the throat or chest, and their shoulders move when they try to breathe deeply. The Hara (energy center) of the human body is located near the navel. It is helpful to try reaching this area with the breath.

Place your hand on your navel, and attempt to breathe deeply into your abdomen. During inhalation, the stomach should move outward, and during exhalation it should retract inward. Breathing deeply helps to circulate the energy more fully around the body. During re-feeding, breathing can help with anxiety associated with eating, as well as provide an energy flow to assist the stomach and intestines in digestion.

Atmosphere

Surround all meals with a peaceful and comfortable atmosphere. Try using candlelight or different colored light bulbs. Place fresh, brightly colored flowers in the center of the table. Play classical music. Use relaxing aromatherapy. Bring out the fancy china and stemware.

Eat in a room of the house besides the kitchen or dining room. Sit in your favorite bean bag chair, or on a fluffy sofa. Eat outside at the picnic table, or on a blanket at the park. Do whatever makes the surroundings more comfortable.

 Have Some Fun!

Adding the element of play can make the process of recovery lighter and easier to cope with. Don't take every moment of life seriously. While preparing food, play some fun music and sing along to it. Purchase a joke book and take turns reading out loud. Watch a video of stand-up comedians. Tell funny stories about childhood. Remember how good it feels to laugh.

Be creative with the food. Try garnishes and vibrant color combinations. Arrange the plate to make a picture. Purchase edible flowers from a specialty market. Use food as a form of artistic expression.

Play restaurant! Create menus with some safe meal choices. Elect a waiter or waitress. Serve the meal in courses.

Much relief can be felt from lightening up.

Talk About Something Else

Another way to make a meal easier is to engage in conversations on subjects other than food and eating. This makes the recovering person feel less paranoid about eating with others. In a family or group setting some simple games may make it easier to direct conversation away from food.

It is important to set ground rules for these activities. Avoid interruptions. Let each person have time to respond, and then move on. Try not to debate what is said. Instead, listen with the intention of learning about each other without judgement or criticism. Encourage participation, but respect each person's right to not respond.

These activities not only divert attention away from food, which makes it easier to eat, but they also help to uncover the true identity, and spark some excitement about the future. Family members or friends may begin to be able to view life through the eyes of others by listening closely to the response given.

Choose a subject and take turns talking about it. Here are some ideas:

1. Talk about a dream you had last night, the best dream you ever had, or the scariest dream you ever had.
2. Tell us about your favorite musician or music group.
3. Describe your favorite animal.
4. Tell us about your favorite movie or book.
5. Describe what a perfect day would be like for you.

Pose a question and give each person a chance to answer. Here are some suggestions:

1. If you could go anywhere on vacation for one week, where would you go, and why?
2. What is your favorite season of the year? Why? What is your least favorite? Why?
3. What do you think God looks like?
4. Who do you think of as a hero? Why?

5.   Do you believe in extra-terrestrial beings?
6.   What do you think is the most important invention of the 20th century?
7.   What do you think will be the most important invention of the 21st century?

What are some other questions or subjects you could suggest?

Positive Affirmations

If you find yourself being trapped by eating-disorder thoughts during the meal, begin reciting positive affirmations between bites of food. The more affirmations are practiced, the more effective they become. You can use activities of the conscious mind, such as affirmations, to reprogram the subconscious mind. It takes consistency of effort to alter the negative internal thought patterns. Even if you don't believe the statements at first, there is some part of you who is listening, and soaking in the praise you deserve.

Here are some affirmation suggestions:

•This food is my friend and partner in healing.

•By choosing to eat this food, I am choosing life over death.

•This food is my medicine.

•Every bite of this food brings me one step closer to reaching my goals and dreams.

•By nourishing my body, I am reclaiming control over my life.

•Eating is a safe and normal part of being human.

•As I eat, I participate in self-care.

•I am beginning a new era of my life; an era filled with possibilities.

•As I nourish myself, the eating disorder becomes weaker, and inner peace becomes a possibility.

• This food feeds the part of me which wants to heal.

•My body accepts this food. It is the helping hand my body needs.

> *"Don't quit when the tide is the lowest, for it is just about to turn. Don't quit over doubts and questions, for there is something you may learn. Don't quit when the night is darkest, for it is just a while 'til dawn. Don't quit when you've run the farthest, for the race is almost won. Don't quit when the hill is steepest, for your goal is almost nigh; Don't quit, for you're not a failure - until you fail to try."*
>
> *-Jill Wolf*

70

•I deserve this meal.

•I deserve to eat.

•I deserve life.

•Each moment I have a choice. I can choose the small and limited world of my eating disorder, or I can choose the vast and colorful world of balance and freedom.

•By letting go of demons, I make room for angels.

•I feel starvation leave my body, and I begin to heal.

•I am proud of my recovery efforts.

•Each day my recovery becomes easier. Each day I come closer to my goal.

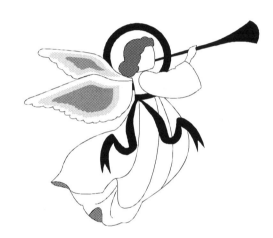

Quieting the Voices

Many people agree that constant negative thoughts are the worst part of having an eating disorder. They try to redirect your determination. However, the thoughts automatically begin to go away if the eating is consistent! The slow and gradual decrease of the voices makes the process of quieting them challenging to endure, but the reward of inner peace is well worth the effort. Imagine an entire hour, or even a whole day, during which you do not worry about food. What relief! Remember, the programs in your brain which feed you self-hatred can be re-formed into programs which feed you self-care. It is only a matter of rearranging your brain's neurons.

"I Can Relate To That!"
Quieting the Voices

I remember sitting in front of my food, and believing I was going to die. My stomach was twisted in knots, and my mind was racing. I felt as if I were being tortured. I was consumed by terrifying thoughts of gaining weight, and how that would affect my life. I thought no one would treat me normally. I was sure these obsessive thoughts about food would be there forever. I was convinced that I was not worthy of having a normal life. I was afraid I would never be able to eat without feeling guilty or thinking I was overweight.

My disorder attacked me with thoughts like:

- You are a big fat pig.
- There will be nothing special about you if you gain weight.
- No one will love you if you gain weight.
- If you eat, you are weak and out of control.
- If you start eating, you won't be able to stop.

It helped to talk out loud about the thoughts in my head. It made them seem less absolute. By sharing my experience with my family, and hearing their views, I learned that my perspective could be altered.

I reached out for support from my family and the support groups. I reminded myself constantly of the goals I wanted to reach. The more meals I was able to eat, the quieter those voices became. Because I had made the decision to recover, I stuck to it. Gradually, the toxic thoughts were defeated by my determination to have my life back.

Retaining Water

Some people retain water in the beginning stages of re-feeding. Do not confuse this with weight gain. It will take anywhere from 4 months to 2 years to reach a healthy body weight. Water retention is especially common among those who abused laxatives or diuretics. It takes time for the body to balance its fluids and electrolytes after being constantly drained. The organs affected, including the kidneys, gall bladder, intestines, and colon, are exhausted from misuse. If laxative abuse continues, the muscles in the colon may permanently relax, which could lead to a loss of control over bowel movements. The body is remarkably able to repair itself, but healing cannot be hurried. You must wait it out, *and continue eating normally*. The water retention will eventually subside. Starting laxative or diuretic use again will make this water retention worse, not to mention threaten your life.

Keeping the Food Down

For those re-feeding after bulimic behavior, keeping the food "down" is the main concern. Your body and mind are used to purging after you eat. It will take courage, patience, and commitment to break this habitual response to a full stomach. Stomach muscles may actually instinctively begin to contract. Anxiety and emotional discharge such as crying or anger are possible as well. The body may become restless.

This section provides helpful hints for keeping food down. Be prepared by reviewing these ideas before every meal, and several times throughout the day. Keep affirmations and a journal nearby. When you look back at these journal entries, you may learn some interesting things about yourself.

Every time you keep the food in your body after eating, you take one step closer to being free of the invader.

*Proclaim today the end of your self-abuse patterns. Promise yourself you are done purging. Remind yourself that you do not want to live this way anymore.

*Promise someone you love that you will not purge anymore. The person can be aware of this promise, but they don't have to be. The person to whom you make the promise can be alive or deceased. This is especially useful when self-esteem is low, and depression is a factor. External motivation can lead to internal motivation.

*Step out of the "just one more time" thoughts, and understand that one more time may be the time you rupture your esophagus and die instantly. Create a collage entitled "Is it worth it?" with photos and statements representing the reasons you want to live (i.e. children, pets, goals, responsibilities, a vacation you have yet to take). Place this collage somewhere between where you eat and where you used to purge; maybe even on the back of the toilet seat.

*Have a plan for after your meals. Decide on an activity before you eat, so you do not have to think about it afterwards. Activities could include: calling a friend, playing with your dog or cat, watching TV, doing artwork, taking a shower, cleaning your house, cleaning the garage, doing yard work, planting flowers, taking a walk, journaling, reading a captivating novel.

*Try to eat with someone who is supportive, and knows about your disorder. Before the meal make a deal! Make it safe for yourself to talk about the feelings you will have during and after the meal. That person can help by reminding you of your goals to heal and be free from bulimia.

*Breathe deeply throughout the entire meal and take your time. The more relaxed your muscles are, the less likely a purge instinct will occur.

*Watch one of your favorite movies while you eat. It may take your attention away from the food, and allow you to finish eating. Then while you continue watching the movie, you can more easily avoid thoughts of purging.

*Journal about the positive experiences you have with not purging. If you have a good day and notice yourself feeling better, write about it. Then, on a challenging day, you can go back and read the positive journal entry, and remind yourself of your abilities to transform.

*Pray! Whatever your beliefs are, faith can be an enormous source of strength during recovery. Ask the deity you recognize for strength and assistance with this struggle.

*Are there people in your life whose motivation and determination you admire? Keep a photograph of them near you as you eat. Try to adopt their use of those remarkable qualities.

The Return Of Hunger

The invader convinced you that you could outsmart hunger; that hunger was just another trick to make you gain weight. The invader saw hunger as the enemy. It demanded that you ignore hunger, and eventually the body understood that sending hunger messages was not working anymore. The body realized it was not being listened to, so the body stopped talking. Its instinctive duty to ask for fuel was turned off.

You will notice as you begin to eat that your hunger will return. The amount of time it takes varies. For some people hunger comes back all at once, and for others it returns gradually. The return of hunger is a wonderful sign that your body is beginning to trust you again. It doesn't have to protect itself from the invader; it can simply ask for what it knows it needs to be healthy.

The return of hunger can be scary, because you are still learning to trust your body. You are gradually beginning to see that your body will only send hunger signals if it needs food. Your body will not trick you into eating to make you overweight. During re-feeding the body may need to ask for food quite often. Every bit of food you ingest is being used immediately to repair all the damage done to the internal organs, bones, and tissues. The amazing body instinctively knows how to heal, as long as it has the right building material, which is food. You must trust that after you have reached a safe weight, the body will adjust hunger to coincide with the new required amount of food. I remember being so hungry that I was afraid I would never stop eating. But eventually my hunger leveled out, and I realized my body had needed all of the food it had asked for to repair itself.

The more you give in to hunger, the faster this process will work. Make a rule for yourself that you will eat whenever you are hungry, regardless of time and place. Promise your body that you will give it what it asks for. Tell your body you trust its ability to ask for the nutrients it needs.

Being Gentle With Your Self

Re-feeding is difficult. It can be exhausting, frustrating, and fear-invoking. There may be days when you feel like giving up. You are not used to caring for yourself. It takes time to learn to accept positive healing vibrations, instead of self-defeating, toxic patterns.

It is extremely beneficial to practice self-nurturing during this time of challenge. You can love yourself in ways that are not related to food or eating. Here are some ideas:

- Bubble baths relieve stress. Try a variety of bath salts, aromatherapy products, and soaps.
- Play a video game, or go to an arcade. This is not only enjoyable, but it can also help your brain begin to function efficiently again.
- Meditate. There are many guided meditation and visualization tapes and books available. Activities like this can help you deepen your breathing and calm anxiety.
- Go outdoors! Take a walk in the woods with a friend, or a pet. Breathe in fresh air. Look at the trees. Connect with Mother Earth.
- Make theme collages: an anger collage, a dream collage, a health collage, etc.
- Write a love poem to yourself. Write all the things you would love to read in the most romantic love poem you can imagine. Hide it in a drawer so you can run across it in the future.

UNPLUG!

The invader needs fuel to survive. Unfortunately, media images, measurements, and scales continually supply that fuel. During recovery, it may be helpful to unplug from influences which support the invader. Backing away from the constant stimulation given by television, magazines, and advertisements can allow a space to grow within you, in which you can begin to form your own ideas about beauty. You have the power to free yourself from the "illusionary-image-prison" created by the collective, low self-esteem of society.

- **JOURNAL BREAK: What Is Beauty?**

- What is beauty to you?

- Try writing a definition of beauty without using any references to physical appearance.

- What qualities make a person beautiful?

- What or who did you think was beautiful when you were a child?

How to Unplug

There are several ways to unplug from detrimental influences. By setting aside low quality, "invader fuel," you make room in the tank for high quality fuel, which will assist you in your healing process. Here are some ways you can unplug:

- Stop watching television. If this seems impossible, start with not watching commercials. Television is full of contradicting messages. Diet advertisements are followed by cheese cake advertisements.   Many popular programs depict an imaginary world, in which value systems are based on fashion and sarcasm. It can be difficult to decipher what is real.

- Stop reading and looking through magazines. The pages of magazines are packed with articles, pictures, and self-tests to prove that there is something wrong with you the way you are, and to sell you the latest product, diet, make-up, or outfit to fix the "problem." Instead, read some inspiring, personal-growth literature, or an exciting adventure novel. Give yourself some high quality fuel. You need new fuel in order to live in a new way.

- Throw away your scale. Regardless of what number appears, the invader will find some way to convince you it is too much. Stop torturing yourself.

- When shopping for new clothes during re-feeding, go with friends. Let them bring you different sizes without you looking at the tags. Choose the clothes that feel most comfortable. After purchasing them, have your friends cut out the size tags. The less you categorize yourself, the more difficult it will be for the invader to find a way in.

- Stop talking about the appearance of others. Stop criticizing the physical form, clothing, or hair of other people. Criticism of others may be a reflection of self-criticism. The less you talk about physical appearance, the less important it will be in your life. In this way, you can free yourself from the invader; for the invader thrives in the competitive world of image.

Why is it important to unplug?

You are in the process of discovering that you are more than your eating disorder. You are finding your self; building a new identity. With many conflicting influences present, it would be easy to replace your eating disorder with another unhealthy coping mechanism. Here is your chance to reach into your core, and change any value systems which support the invader. Replace them with values which support the person you are becoming; free from the invader's grasp. Until you do this, the invader will find a way in. If not through food, through some other method of self-destruction. By unplugging you deny the invader what it needs to survive within you, and it will have no choice but to retreat.

JOURNAL BREAK: New Fuel

- How could you unplug from toxic fuel in your life?

- What activities or images could you adopt, which would offer you a higher quality fuel?

As You Heal

Re-feeding is the perfect process to help you believe in yourself. After traveling this rocky road, you will look back and pat yourself on the back for making it through the tough days. You will be amazed at your own strength. You will feel a new confidence building within. It takes a powerful person to transform a lifestyle from one of destruction to one of healing.

As you become healthier, you will notice subtle changes in your life. You may find it easier to understand things you read. You may feel your depression lifting. You may catch yourself dreaming about your future. You may smile more often. You may not need to sleep as much, or you may need to sleep more. You may feel anxious to go out into the world and live! Let your unique process unfold, and document it along the way.

On-going Journal Exercises
Purchase a journal specifically for daily re-feeding exercises.

1. Each day write about the feelings which surfaced during meals. Was it difficult to keep the food down? Was eating easier or more difficult than the day before? What did you do that helped? What could you do next time?
2. What was happening in your relationships with family, friends, and co-workers throughout the day? Did the status of your relationships help or hinder your ability to eat?
3. Did you notice any changes in energy level, mood, or mental clarity?
4. Did you notice any physical changes (hot flashes, hunger pains, headaches, fatigue)?

SELF-CHECK
Shade in how much of you is still controlled by the eating disorder.

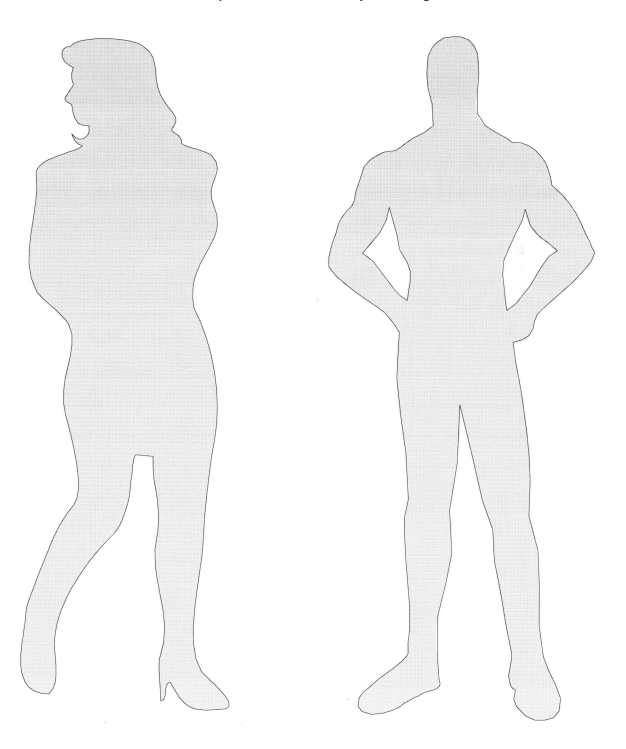

Chapter Seven

Emotions: The Rescue Mission

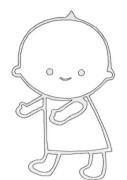

Your Natural State

You are born into the world completely amazed with life, thrilled with the discovery of your toes and fingers, and delighted with the sound of your own voice. You arrive in love with yourself and everything around you. You are not self-conscious about your body. You do not compare yourself to other babies. You do not doubt your own greatness. You are a miracle. You are full of love and cheer. That is your natural state; and if love is your natural state, everything that is not love must be unnatural. You have to be taught how to be unnatural. You have to *learn* how to dislike yourself, criticize yourself, and abuse yourself; for it is unnatural. It is a program you learn in order to cope with anything that feels painful: emotionally, physically, and psychologically. With each painful circumstance, harsh word, and incomprehensible wound, your self-love is gradually covered by self-protective mechanisms. It hurts not to be able to be natural, not to be able to be yourself. Something must be wrong. You must adjust, or live in pain and confusion. To stop the pain, you shut down your natural state. It hurts too much to be pulled back and forth. It hurts too much to be different, and so you become like everyone else.

The Invader's Garden Of Weeds

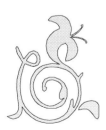

You eventually center yourself where everyone in your environment is centered - the invader's garden of weeds. In this garden, the invader infects every seed with the lie: "There is something wrong with you."

Growing up in this garden, you forget all about your true nature of love. You learn to value your worldly accomplishments, instead of your inherent qualities. You learn to be hard on yourself, criticize yourself, and punish yourself. You are shown guilt, shame, and disappointment. You are told that some people are prettier, smarter, or more talented than other people. You are taught that loving yourself means you are conceited. You begin to categorize everyone. You find that no one is good enough; that something is wrong with everyone. You stop being delighted with life. Eventually, you learn how to switch off your feelings, because it hurts too much to feel; and this is where you live. This is your world. Joy and love, the very state in which you entered the world, is hidden away in the depths of your being.

The Rescue Mission

Love is the force strong enough to dig you out of the invader's weed garden and re-plant you in the lush fields of life! The invader fertilizes you with fear to make you think you are not capable of living outside of the garden of weeds. It feeds you "weed food." But you are not a weed! You are a beautiful, blooming, bright flower. It is time to cut away the gnarly vines of the invader's weed garden. It is time to climb out of the lifeless muck in which you are trapped. It is time to dig deep into the soil and rescue the seed within you that was infected long ago. It is time to wipe away the lies and uncover the truth: there is ***nothing*** wrong with you.

All of the strength you need for recovery is confined within your emotional self which has been locked up by the invader. It is time to free the hostages. It is time to claim what is rightfully yours. It is time to rediscover the magic of your existence, and be once again delighted with life. It is time to rewrite the program that has been running your life.

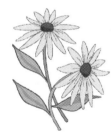

JOURNAL BREAK: Create Your Garden
1. Draw a picture or write a description of the garden in which you would choose to grow if you were a flower. What type of flower are you? Are there butterflies in your garden? Where is your garden? Is the sun shining?

2. Plant some new seeds in your garden to replace the old seeds which were tainted by the invader. What are some healthy ideas on which you would like your life to be based?

The Color Of Life

Emotions are the color of life. They are the dance of the heart, constantly moving in diverse and wonderful patterns. Emotions motivate all action. They inspire us, compel us, awaken us. When emotions are intense, they can motivate us to accomplish the impossible. Emotions are the force behind all change.

The invader convinces you that only a black and white world exists, and that this color is not for you. It tells you that you do not deserve color, are not worthy of color, and won't ever find color. But the invader is lying! It is lying to you to keep you from escaping the garden of weeds. Claim the color! Claim your color! Stop treating yourself as though you are a weed in a black and white world.

ACTIVITY BREAK: Breathing In Color

Color is one of the ways emotions communicate. Using crayons, colored pencils, or chalk, fill in each square with a different color. Then label each square with the emotion you feel is accurately represented by that color.

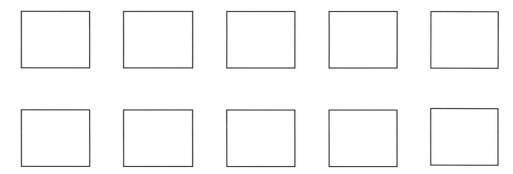

Giving these emotions a color creates a symbol which you can use to help make experiencing these emotions a little easier. Use this exercise whenever you feel overwhelmed by an emotion.

Sit comfortably and draw some deep breaths into your stomach. Close your eyes and imagine the air you are breathing to be the color of the emotion you would *like* to be feeling at the moment. With each exhalation, visualize the color of the undesirable emotion flowing out of your body. With every inhalation, visualize the color of your desired emotional state flowing into your body. For example: Perhaps I am feeling jealousy (green), and I want to feel joy (yellow). I would picture the air flowing into my body as yellow, and the air flowing out of my body as green.

This exercise in and of itself may not completely process the emotions being felt, but it can be a helpful coping tool.

Negative Or Toxic?

There is space within you for every emotion, positive and negative. Negative emotions are equally as valid as positive emotions. Sadness and crying are just as cleansing to the emotional self as laughter and joy. Unfortunately, we live in a society which often denies the presence of negative emotions, and tries to avoid them. Negative emotions are labeled as "bad" or "weak." This can lead to those emotions becoming toxic.

When an emotion is labeled as "bad", and is stifled or unexpressed, that emotion is pushed into the shadows of your being. Every time that emotion is triggered, the stifling is repeated. Through life, all of this unexpressed emotional energy accumulates and begins to overflow. As that emotion is *not allowed to be*, it becomes *toxic*. There is nowhere for this mound of raw emotion to hide, and since energy can neither be created nor destroyed (according to the first law of thermodynamics), it finds some way to express itself in one's life; perhaps through a disease, a self-destructive habit, or the abuse of others.

Remember what you read in Chapter Two: Understanding the Invader. During phase one, the invader takes the negative emotions as prisoners to use against you later, and lets you believe you are joyful and happy since you are controlling your food intake. This is how the invader keeps hold of you. When you start to experience uncomfortable feeling states, it makes you think that your eating disorder is the only way to express those hidden, dark emotions that have become toxic, and are eating you away inside. It intensifies anger, depression, and fear by adding shame and guilt to the mixture. The invader keeps you consumed in your own shadow, convincing you that you do not deserve to live in the light. But the light is your natural state of being, and it includes negative emotions. You need only redefine the emotions you have avoided feeling for so long, and gradually reintegrate them.

JOURNAL BREAK: Finding the light side of negative emotions
Answer the following questions in relation to each of the emotions listed below.
- How could the negative emotion be useful in your life? (For example: Anger can serve as a powerful motivator for change.)
- What would be a healthy way to express the negative emotion? (For example: I could redirect the energy that comes with anger toward my efforts of changing my life for the better. When I feel like giving up, I can use the anger to remind myself of what the invader has cost me in my life. The anger can serve as fuel to continue fighting for my life.)
- Write or draw a situation in which these emotions would be appropriate when expressed in a healthy way.

Sadness:

Depression:

Anger:

Fear:

Loneliness:

What are some other negative emotions?

Giving Yourself Permission

An important part of recovery is to give yourself permission to feel what you are

> *Every day is brand new, with no mistakes in it!*
> -Anne Shirley
> *Anne of Green Gables*

feeling, regardless of how painful or joyous it may be. Part of self-care is learning to allow yourself to be yourself, without criticism. If the expression of feelings is avoided, those feelings become a weight attached to you, dragging behind you. This weight becomes heavier and bigger as you drag it. The bigger it grows, the more ashamed you are of it, and the shame piles on top of it. This makes it even heavier, and more difficult to hide. Soon, you cannot move because this weight is so heavy. If you do not give yourself permission to fully feel each moment, you become stuck. If all of your energy is being directed toward fixing what was wrong with yesterday, how can you fully experience today?

Giving yourself permission to fully feel each moment, and then to move through it, does not mean you cannot change. Quite the contrary! It is the only way you *can* truly change. Severing yourself from the limitations of yesterday gives you the freedom to choose who you want to be today. With no unfinished emotional business in yesterday, you have a clean slate for today. Stop trying to fix the past. By trying to fix the past, you keep it in the present. Live today how you want to live today. Forget about how you lived yesterday. In every moment, you have the power to choose.

Giving yourself permission to feel can be scary. Eating disorders can cause emotions to become numb. You are not used to feeling! You do not know what to do with the emotional energy. Your emotional digestion has ceased along with your physical digestion. Anger, frustration, fear, guilt, shame, sadness, and worry can be overwhelming when your old way of coping is no longer available. This is why it is so important to let yourself experience the emotion, and then move through it. Find what is on the other side of those tears. Dive into that state, and find what is hidden beneath it. Push through! Let it out! Your strength may be buried beneath your sadness. Your motivation may be buried under your anger. Your self-love may be hidden behind your shame. Your courage may be concealed by your fear.

This Is Normal!

It is normal to experience emotional discomfort during re-feeding. The emotions are linked to the physical body. As the body begins to wake up, so will your feelings. You are remembering *how to feel*. You may not be able to control them at first, but it will eventually come into a harmonious balance. You have to let them out in order for them to be reorganized in a healthy and manageable way. You may find yourself laughing or crying for no apparent reason. You may experience intense sadness or anger about injustice in society or environmental destruction. You may feel the weight of the entire world's problems on your shoulders. ***This is all normal.*** You are releasing a bulk of raw emotion which has been accumulating for a long time. Let it out so you can be free.

Digest the feelings. If emotions continue to be stifled, they harden into a kind of prison. This prison holds you back. This prison keeps you in cycles which do not serve your best interest. Break out of that prison! Unlock the door and push through the discomfort. This is the only way to reach the freedom of balance. The excess must be released. Then you can sort it out, decide what to reintegrate, and what to transform. Dig through the crust of the invader into the rich soil of your true self. In this soil, new seeds can be planted. In this soil, new dreams can be reached. In this soil, all limits disappear.

JOURNAL BREAK: How Do You Feel?

While living inside of an eating disorder, emotions become numb. You actually forget *how to feel*. It is time to rescue what was held hostage by the invader. It is time to reclaim your power. It is time to remember how to feel.

1. Go outside and look around. Notice the trees, the grass, the flowers, the clouds in the sky, the snow, the rain. Listen to the sounds. Breathe in the scents around you. Take some deep breaths and let yourself feel what you are taking in from nature. What emotions surface when you relax and absorb these natural impressions?

2. Through words, collage work, or an illustration, describe what "the depths of despair" are for you. What situations or memories take you there?

3. Write or draw about something that inspires passion in you.

4. What are you most afraid of? Why?

5. Describe a time in your life when you felt filled with rage.

6. When was the last time you felt happy?

How an Emotion Becomes a Weed

When one emotion is given too much energy, it begins to leak into other emotions, causing them to malfunction. For example, if fear has overgrown into anger and sadness, these emotions may be mixed together, causing confusion. A person may feel angry, but it may just be fear hiding behind rage. A person may feel depressed, but it may just be fear hiding behind sadness. The overgrown emotion does everything it can not to be seen. If it is exposed, it will lose some of its control, its territory, its power. The overgrown emotion begins to cloud the emotions it bleeds upon. Those emotions then function within the shadow of the emotion which is overtaking them.

The way to begin equalizing the emotions is to observe them. Start to know your feelings. Where do they come from? What emotions are stifled or have been stifled throughout your life?

JOURNAL BREAK: Take a look!
When you feel an intense emotion rising within you, go somewhere quiet and take a closer look at it. Write or draw in your journal about what you are feeling. Try answering these questions in relation to your emotional state:

1. What person, memory, circumstance, song, scent, or sight triggered this emotion?

2. What color is the emotion you are feeling?

3. What would you call the emotion you are feeling?

4. Is it possible that a different emotion is present, behind the one mentioned? Could this overgrown emotion be taking up too much space in your feeling self?

5. Are you comfortable with this emotion?

6. How can you express this emotion in a healthy way?

The Fear Monster

It stands behind you. It follows you everywhere. It whispers in your ear. It tells you that everyone is looking at you, judging you, criticizing you. It tells you that no one likes you, and that no one cares about you. It tells you that you are not good enough; not strong enough. It tells you that you cannot recover. It tells you not to try, because you might fail. It tells you that you have to lie to cover up all of your imperfections. It tells you to settle for less than you deserve. It tells you that someone is going to hurt you if you allow yourself to love. It tells you to play it safe, not take risks, follow the crowd. It tells you not to trust anyone. It tells you that you can't reach your dreams, so you might as well not try. It tells you not to live, because living is too scary! ***This lying, life-stealing voice is the fear monster!***

The fear monster is the invader's best friend. You feed the fear monster every time you don't say something you want to say, or don't do something you want to do, because you are afraid. The fear monster feeds on your fear. The larger the fear monster grows, the more difficult it becomes to overcome fear. Everyone has fear, and in some instances, this emotion is appropriate. But if fear grows too large, it will start to make decisions for you, and your power to choose dwindles.

The only way to shrink the fear monster is with courage. Do exactly what terrifies you! By pushing through the fear monster's barrier, you reclaim that energy you had been giving away. When you do this, you will feel a rush of energy fill your body. You will feel the strength gained from facing your fears.

In every moment, you have the choice. Would you rather feed the fear monster, or your courage? Would you rather give away your energy, or cultivate it within you and use it to reach your every dream? Would you rather travel the road the fear monster chooses, or the road of self-care and healing?

JOURNAL/ACTIVITY BREAK: Identify Your Fear Monster

Expose the lie of the fear monster! Drag it out of the shadows and into the light. It won't show itself easily. It will try to hide. It is a living thing that has attached itself to you, and it will fight for its existence. An important part of taking your power back from the fear monster is being able to recognize it. Only then can you begin to know when you are being controlled by the fear monster, and when you are standing in your truth.

- What does your fear monster's voice sound like? Describe the tone it uses with you. Is it sly and manipulative? Is it harsh and crass? How does it try to convince you that it is your voice you are hearing, and not the fear monster's?

- What does your fear monster say to you? What words does it use to convince you to be afraid instead of brave? Does it tell you that no one will like you if you show your true self? Does it tell you that no one will understand if you talk about your feelings?

- What does your fear monster look like? Draw or find a picture of it. Is it ghoulish and creepy? Does it have fangs? Be graphic. It helps to have an actual image of what you are up against.

- What are some things that the fear monster has kept you from achieving?

- How could you reclaim your power from the fear monster?

- How does the fear monster affect your recovery?

The Invader's Thugs: Shame and Guilt

Just when you think you are out of the invader's grasp, the invader pulls out its serious arsenal. It can feel that you are becoming stronger, and that you can no longer be fooled by the usual lies. Sending out its thugs, Guilt and Shame, is the invader's last chance at keeping you in its thrall.

Guilt and Shame attack when you least expect it. You might find yourself feeling especially strong one day, and out of nowhere will come one of these thoughts:

- You don't deserve to get better.
- You should feel embarrassed about your eating disorder.
- You make everyone miserable; everyone would be happier without you.
- Look what you did to yourself.
- Everyone is tired of hearing about your struggle.
- If you haven't recovered by now, you aren't going to.
- You should be ashamed of yourself.
- Its too late now, you have ruined your life. You can never rebuild all that you have lost. You'll never have those opportunities again, even if you do recover.

These are all lies. Don't be fooled! That is not you talking! It is Guilt and Shame. They will stoop lower than low in order to lure you back into the invader's grasp. They will try to make you feel guilty about what you have done to your body, how you have affected your family and friends, the opportunities you missed, and anything else that might weaken you. Guilt and Shame will even try to inspire self-criticism about things completely unrelated to your eating disorder. Suddenly you will find yourself feeling guilty about everything. The mission of Guilt and Shame is to make you feel so bad about yourself that you will give up on living, and turn back to the invader. They will try to make you doubt all the work you are putting into healing. They will try to convince you that you truly are a weed instead of a flower, and that you belong in the garden of weeds.

However, there is a flaw in Guilt and Shame's system. Guilt and Shame use guilt and shame to make you do exactly what they tell you to feel guilty and ashamed about. For instance, they guilt and shame you into eating disorder behavior, then they make you feel guilty and ashamed of your disorder, and then they finish by making you feel guilty and ashamed about feeling guilty and ashamed. It is a vicious cycle. There is no way to please them. If you listen to Guilt and Shame, you will never feel anything except guilt and shame. Why would you want to continue the very behavior for which they are attacking you?

This illogical system of guilt and shame is another way to prove that the invader is simply an overgrown lie. The invader force feeds you low quality weed food (like guilt and shame) in order to trap you in the garden of weeds. But you are a flower, and weed food will not help you grow. All the weed food in the world cannot keep you from pushing past the invader's thugs, and replanting yourself into your true, life-filled, flower garden.

JOURNAL BREAK: Identify Guilt and Shame

- What do your Guilt and Shame thugs look like? Cut and paste, or draw a picture of them, in the boxes below. Personifying Guilt and Shame will help you recognize them. Also, separating yourself from Guilt and Shame can grant you the relief of knowing that *those voices are not your true voice*. Guilt and Shame are just more of the invader's tricks to keep you down. Their voices may have a different tone inside of your head. They may become stronger when you are near certain people. What do they sound like? What do they say to you? Do they feed you weed food? What do they try to make you feel guilty or ashamed about? Are you going to let these two thugs stand in your way? Talk to them as if they were real people standing in front of you. Tell them to get out of your way, you have work to do!

Guilt

Shame

Dissolving Guilt and Shame

After identifying Guilt and Shame, and separating them from your self, there are active things you can do to dissolve their influence in your life.

- Openly tell someone something Shame is trying to make you feel ashamed about. For example, tell others who are unaware of your eating disorder about your struggle. Watch the reaction. More than likely, they will express concern and relief that you have confided in them. I was astonished at how my shame disappeared as I became more open about what I was going through. Shame had tried to convince me that people in this world are harsh and judgmental. But every time I pushed Shame aside and shared my experience, people responded in a warm and caring way. As I followed Shame's lead less and less, its influence on my life dwindled.

- Make a list of every person whom you feel you have affected negatively with your eating disorder. Call or speak with each one. Tell them you are trying to overcome the guilt associated with your disorder. Ask them for help. Tell them you feel guilty about having affected them. I predict that no one would respond with, "I want you to feel guilty for having an eating disorder and affecting my life so drastically." Instead, they probably just want to see you happy and well. We must learn to see that Guilt is just one of the invader's lies. It only exists if we believe it.

- Put down the "should stick." The "should stick" is just something we beat ourselves with. It has no other purpose. Every time you say, "I should have done this," or, "I shouldn't have done this," or, "I should be better," you are beating yourself. Put down that should stick. Take that word "should" out of your vocabulary. Stop beating yourself. The "should stick" is incapable of empowering you. It is incapable of lifting you up. It is incapable of helping you escape the invader. The "should stick" is one of Guilt and Shame's most frequently utilized weapons. They hand it to you, and you beat yourself with it. Put it down. Give it back to them and send them on their way.

- Stop apologizing! Don't be sorry about anything. This does not mean that you avoid responsibility for your actions. It simply means you trust the process of life. If you are constantly apologizing for your actions, words, feelings - for your self in general, you end up actually apologizing for your existence. Then Guilt and Shame show up to reinforce that idea, by telling you to feel guilty about being alive, or needing to eat, or to feel ashamed of yourself for taking up space in the world. Being sorry is just an open door for Guilt and Shame to come in and steal your power.

The Secret Weapon

As you come closer to rescuing your emotions, and pushing the invader out of your life, the invader will strengthen its forces to try to prevent your escape. It knows that once you re-integrate emotional power into your life, it has no chance of keeping you in the garden of weeds. The invader will use Guilt, Shame, and the fear monster to wear you down. At times, self-doubt will be so prevalent you may think you are incapable of making decisions. On some days, depression will seem so unbearable that you might want to give up. However, you, the warrior fighting for your life, have a secret weapon. This secret weapon is the only force strong enough to overcome and dissolve fear. This secret weapon is the only force big enough to push the invader out of your life forever. This secret weapon is the only force capable of pulling you out of those days when voices such as, "You can't do it," and, "You're not good enough," are screaming at you inside of your head. This secret weapon is sharp enough to cut back the gnarly vines of the invader's garden of weeds, and open up the path to your rightful place in the sun. This secret weapon will save you, lift you up, empower you, and never let you down - if you use it. The secret weapon is:

ACTIVE SELF-LOVE

Do Something!

You have heard over and over that you have to love yourself; that loving yourself comes first before you can love anyone else. This is true, but how do you do it? What can you actively do to love yourself? How do you train your brain to feed you loving thoughts instead of self-defeating thoughts? How do you change behaviors that hurt you? How do you change the deeply ingrained belief that something is wrong with you? *You must be active*! You must *do* something different in order to achieve different results.

Just reading this book, without implementing any of the ideas in it, will do you no good. You must do the activities, even when they feel uncomfortable - *especially* when they feel uncomfortable. That discomfort is the breaking down of an out-of-date, useless behavior pattern. That breaking down is essential for the success of constructing a new way of living.

Live in Love

Actively love yourself. Fill your days with activities which support your recovery. Don't give your energy to anything else while you are healing. Make your healing process the focus of your every moment. In doing this, you won't leave any spaces through which the invader, the fear monster, or Guilt and Shame could sneak.

- Say the affirmations even when you don't believe them.
- Make collages or affirmation signs every day and hang them around your house.
- Carry your journal with you everywhere, and journal about thoughts, feelings and experiences throughout the day.
- Set a timer to go off every fifteen minutes. Every time it goes off, ask yourself the following questions:

    1.Am I actively loving myself?

    2.If not, how can I actively love myself, right now?

- Make a list of ways you can love yourself. The list could consist of loving thoughts (flower food) and actions; replacements for self-defeating, fear thoughts (weed food).
- Listen to affirmation, meditation, relaxation, or self-esteem tapes while you drive, clean the house, or prepare meals.
- Go to support groups.
- Spend time with people who feed the part of you which wants to be well.
- Write a story. Create a character. Make up a story out of your imagination. It doesn't have to make sense. Just let your mind flow.
- Tape pictures on your wall of people you admire. Remind yourself of how powerful one human being can be.
- Go to church, meditate, read sacred text, or take a spirituality class of some kind. Feed your spirit with higher ideas. Remind yourself that you are more than just your body.
- Rent your favorite funny movie, remember how it feels to laugh.
- Invite some friends over and play a board game. Participate in life.
- Plant some flowers in your yard. As you care for them, imagine that you are nurturing and growing the new, healthy seeds within you. Actually create the flower garden in which you would like to grow up.
- Rent or purchase a book of love poems and read them aloud to yourself. Even if it feels silly at first, a part of you is listening who needs to hear those kind words.
- Speak to yourself kindly. Practice being gentle with yourself. Compliment yourself. Every day, think of some area of life in which you are competent. Pat yourself on the back. If it helps, imagine you are speaking to a little child inside of you. When you catch yourself being critical of yourself, ask yourself this question: "Would I speak to a child in this way? How would hearing these words affect a child?"

When you actively love yourself, you don't have time to do anything else. You don't have time to doubt yourself, criticize yourself, or feel ashamed of yourself. When you fill your days with active self-love, you leave no space for self-hate. And, best of all, when you practice constant self-love - you allow yourself to grow. Have you ever known anything to grow without love of some kind? Plants only grow when they receive love in the form of rain and sunshine. Children only grow when they are held, fed, and nurtured. You will only grow beyond this challenge if you provide the love and nurturing you need. Breathe love, speak love, think love, and feel love. Let this secret weapon permeate every moment of every day - and you will be free. Free, and once again in your natural state. Amazed by the miracle of life. Delighted by the magic of your existence.

CHAPTER EIGHT

The House of Being

The House of Being

How do you identify yourself? What are you made of? Are you only flesh and blood? Where does your personality come from? Where are emotions produced? Where are thoughts processed? What would you term the totality which is you? I call it your House of Being - the thoughts, emotions, intuitions, talents, body, personality, spirit, and all other attributes of which you consist. All that you are is your House of Being.

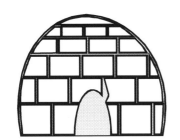

Many people walk through life without considering this idea. All that you are is not contained only within your physical body. All of your components, including your physical body, make up a unified whole. And you have the ability, the opportunity, and the privilege to explore, examine, redecorate, redefine, reorganize, rebuild, appreciate, express, and fully utilize every room within your unified whole; your House of Being. By investing time and effort in the development of each room, the efficiency and productivity of the entire house improves.

The physical body is one room in your house of being. It is an integral part of the whole. The better it functions, the higher the quality of contribution it offers to your entirety. The key is finding the balance. There is an appropriate level of quality care for the physical body. There is also an appropriate level of healthy discipline. The wise master of the House of Being strikes a balance.

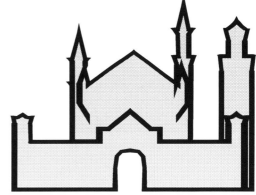

The physical form is extremely important. But there is more to you! If all of your energy is put into maintaining, altering, examining, criticizing, and trying to fix your physical body, there is not much energy left for managing the other rooms. The body begins to be blamed for everything which goes wrong in all of the other rooms (emotional life, professional life, intellectual life, family life), and even more energy is given to the body to attempt to remedy the problem. But the real problem is: There is no way to repair these other rooms by continuing to rearrange the body room. The body room must be carefully put back into place, and then the rest of the house can receive the attention it rightly deserves.

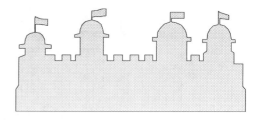

ACTIVITY BREAK: Create Your House of Being

- What does your House of Being look like? Is it a castle, a mansion, an igloo, a country house on a hill? What color(s) is it? Describe your House of Being with a drawing or through words, or find a picture of your House of Being and paste it in the space below.

- What is in your House of Being? What rooms are on the first floor? The second? What is in the basement? The attic?

- On what floor is your physical body?

- Is the light on in every room? Which rooms are dark? Which rooms are cluttered and need some attention? Which rooms are neat and organized? Which rooms need some redecorating?

- On which floor do you spend most of your time? In which room? Why?

Live In Your House of Being

After you create your house of being - live there! If you remain in your house of being, you will not be as affected by the external happenings of the world, and you will not be as focused on your body. You will begin to spend time in the other rooms, and realize how much more there is to you than you once thought.

Consider the following tale:

> *A powerful warlord built up his army, and conquered a nearby city. He ordered everyone to evacuate his newly claimed territory. Anyone who did not comply was killed. His army went through the city, burning homes, and pushing the people off their land.*
>
> *As the warlord walked through the city, assessing his new acquisition, he came upon a monastery, and went inside. He found a monk, sitting quietly in meditation. He walked up to the monk, enraged that he was not following the evacuation order.*
>
> *"This is my city now! Be gone!" screamed the warlord. But the monk did not move.*
>
> *"Have you no idea that you are looking at a man who will slice you in two with this sword without batting an eyelash?" he threatened, raising his sword.*
>
> *The monk calmly replied, "Have you no idea that you stand before a man who could let you do exactly that without batting an eyelash?"*

- Where did the monk live?

The Invitation

Many people with eating disorders see the body as something outside of the self; something that needs to be fixed or altered. It is kept on the outskirts, in the yard, tied up to the fence. It is exiled and abandoned. Because of this illusion of separateness from the body, suffering occurs. It is time to invite the body back into the House of Being, where it belongs. Break down the walls of inner-separation. Welcome your body into your totality. Claim it as yours. It is the only one you have, and it is in your care right now.

The Invitation

I, _____, humbly invite my body back into my House of Being. I acknowledge my body as an important part of who I am.

I am grateful for my body, for it allows me to be here. I am committed to helping my body heal the wounds it incurred during its time in exile, so that it may produce the energy it is designed to produce.

I claim my body, and take full responsibility for its well being. I will be gentle with my body, I will give my body what it needs, and I will not overwork my body. I will no longer treat my body as something which needs to be altered of fixed. Instead, I will accept my body exactly as it is, and thank it for giving me another chance.

I open the door, and I welcome my body home, back to my House of Being.

Signed:_____

Date:_____

Witness:_____

Date:_____

Home Maintenance

As you expand your idea of "you" to accommodate your House of Being instead of only your physical body, some new ideas regarding self-care may become applicable. You may want to consider expanding your definition of "food." There are many different kinds of food. Physical food for the physical body is only one kind of food.

There is also:
- Emotional food
- Thought food
- Impression food
- Interactive food

Part of home maintenance is choosing a higher quality of each of these foods. It is similar to gasoline in automobiles. A car runs more efficiently, and lasts longer, if it receives high grade gasoline, is kept clean, and if the oil is changed on a regular basis.

Emotional Food

What feelings are you feeling? Emotions feed your emotional self, which is a room in your house of being. Emotions communicate through color, music, and plants. Look at your living space, your car, your wardrobe. Maybe it is time to wear some new colors or buy some new house plants? Plant a new tree in your backyard. Plant a vegetable garden. Buy yourself some flowers. Start listening to a wonderful new radio station, or buy some new compact discs. What are some ways you could freshen up the your emotional self with some higher quality emotional food?

Thought Food

What thoughts are you thinking? Thoughts feed your intellectual self. The invader feeds you low-quality thought food in the form of negative self-talk. Maybe its time to buy or rent some new books. Listen to a book on tape while you drive. Go to a poetry reading. Feed your intellectual self with some invigorating ideas. What have you always been curious about? Start reading about that. Take a class in a subject you have never studied before. What are some other forms of higher quality thought food?

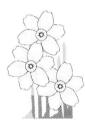

Impression Food

What do your surroundings look like? What do they smell like? What you see and smell can dramatically alter your mood. When you look around at your living space, do you like what you see? What changes would you like to make? Perhaps you could paint your walls, move around your furniture, light some incense, burn candles, put a new picture on the mantle, buy some fresh flowers for every room, organize a closet, throw away things you do not need. Spend some time outdoors. Go to a local state park and take a walk in the woods. Breathe different air. Look at different sights. Drive on a road you have never driven before. Clean out the garage. Trim the bushes. Wash the floors. Give yourself some new impressions. You are reforming your internal self, so it seems appropriate to adjust your external surroundings. You may find your tastes changing as you change. What are some ideas you have for changing the impressional food in your surroundings?

Interactive Food

With whom are you spending time? Do they support your healing process? Do they speak to you with kindness? Who in your life makes you laugh? Do you need to distance yourself from some toxic relationships? Spend time with a healthy support network. Go to church if it helps. Attend a support group at a local hospital. Give your interactive self some fresh food by creating new and interesting relationships. Can you think of some new, healthy interactive food you could incorporate into your life?

Home Security

Your House of Being is your responsibility, so you must not only care for it, but also protect it by making safe and healthy choices for yourself. This is another part of self-care. You have the ability to decide what you let into and out of your House of Being. You can use discretion when choosing what food (of all types) to accept and what food to bypass. This is what I call "home security." Here are some ways to practice home security:

- Put solid "locks" on your "doors." Keep the "keys" in a safe place, and do not give them away. If your House of Being is locked, and you are the only one who has the keys, then you are the only one who can decide who and what enters your House of Being. Only you decide who you see, talk to, and spend time with. This also applies to media exposure. Make a conscious decision about what you are watching on television and at the movies. What are you letting into your House of Being? How are you being influenced by your media exposure? This may be a good time to stop watching commercials which may trigger your eating disorder thoughts. It may be a good idea to rent comedic or inspirational films, instead of heavy personal dramas or intense historical epics. Try listening to music which is uplifting or relaxing rather than angry or sarcastic. What you are taking in affects you in more ways than you realize. Filter it!
- Implement an inner alarm system. Notice your triggers. What people, situations, or locations instigate eating disorder behavior in you? Pay attention to what happens in your physical body when you are having a challenging moment. Maybe your stomach

tenses up. Maybe you have a headache, or become quiet. Perhaps you hide in your room. Watch for your habits and document them. This can be your alarm system. When you begin to feel one of those responses building, you can recognize it and take action to change your course. You can learn to trust yourself by listening to your body responses. You will know when something "doesn't feel right," and then you have the power to choose differently, and protect your House of Being.

Building Sovereignty: Active Empowerment

You can build the integrity and sovereignty of your House of Being by actively empowering yourself.

Strong Words

One way to do this is to put the power back into your words. What you say strongly affects how you feel and think.

Here are some examples:

- Instead of saying, "I'll try," say, "**I will!**"
- Instead of saying, "I hope things change for me," say, "**I am going** to change things in my life."
- Instead of saying, "I can't believe it," say, "I **can** believe it!"

Rework some sentences. How could you put more power into what you are saying? What could you say instead of "maybe," or, "I guess so," or "I don't know?"

> *"Whether you say you can, or you say you can't - you're right!"*
> **-Henry Ford**

Tell the Truth

Stop lying! Even the little ones hurt you inside. When we lie, we are attempting to cover up those things about us that we think are "wrong." But there is nothing wrong with you. There is no reason to lie. When somebody asks you how you are, tell them the truth. If you feel terrific, say so; if not, say so. Share yourself! Be responsible for your words. When you make a promise, keep it. Say what you mean, and mean what you say. Telling the truth not only fights off Shame, but it raises your self-esteem as well. The invader makes us think we have to lie in order to cover up all of our faults. Lying is food for the invader. The truth *shall* set you free. It is a great feeling to tell the truth, and notice the profound difference it makes in your life.

Do Things On Your Own

Set small goals for yourself. Choose a few small projects you would like to begin and complete by yourself. Doing things on your own is a great way to build self-confidence. Here are some ideas:

- Build something.
- Learn a craft, like beading or sewing.
- Take a day trip.
- Do a book report.
- Clean out your closet.
- Plant some flowers.
- Write a short story.
- Go to a local park and pick up garbage.
- Do something nice for your grandparents.
- Volunteer at a nursing home or an animal shelter.
- Install a shelf on the wall.
- Start a scrapbook.
- Memorize the periodic table of elements.
- Take a Tai Chi or yoga class.
- Make a family tree.
- Paint your room a new color.

Connect With Something Greater

Perhaps the most important part of healing the House of Being is establishing a connection with something greater than yourself. That "something greater" is different for everyone. For some it may be God, for others, Great Spirit, Mother Earth and Father Sky, or Great Other Dimension (G.O.D.). For some, it may be Buddha, Jesus, or Ammachi. It may be simply the idea of complete peace, or pure, unconditional love. Some may think of it as where they come from. Others may think of it as where they are going. Some may see it as the Creator of life, the meaning of life, or the reason for life.

Regardless of the name you choose, the description you offer, or the entity you recognize, the connection is what is important. This connection is what will hold you up when no human interaction seems to help. It will be the sunshine on your cloudy day. It will remind you how blessed you are just to be alive. It will support and love you unconditionally. The stronger this connection, the stronger you become. There are many ways to find, maintain, and build upon a connection with something greater than yourself. Here are just a few ideas:

- Pray. Prayer is one of the most powerful tools available. Enter into dialog with whatever God you recognize. There is no right or wrong way to pray. Sing out loud. Write it down. Kneel beside the bed. Go outside and talk to the sky. Talk while you drive, or while you cook. Imagine a divine friend there beside you, listening intently to every word.

- Visit a church. Perhaps you are already a member of a congregation. Perhaps you could try some new churches. Whatever feels comfortable is just fine. There is something powerful about ritual.
- Read books. There are many sacred texts available from several different religious traditions. Read the one(s) with which you resonate. The words in sacred lore have a higher, healing vibration. (There are some suggestions in the Book Suggestion List at the end of the book.)
- Spend time outdoors. Find a place in the woods you like to visit. Make it your special place. Bring special stones there and make a formation on the ground. The earth is extremely powerful. Making an earth connection can be soothing, comforting, and healing.

Your House of Being is who you are. It is more than your body, more than your illness, more than your habits, more than your past. Your full potential exists within your House of Being. It is all within reach. You need only do the exploration, organization, and development. Take the time to learn about yourself, know yourself, and care for yourself. The self-love you will cultivate deep within yourself cannot be touched by the invader.

SELF-CHECK

Shade in how much of you is still controlled by the eating disorder. Is it changing?

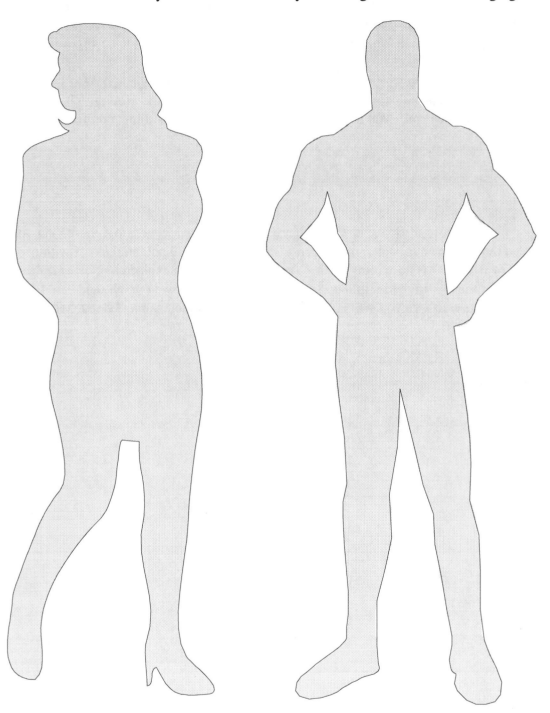

CHAPTER NINE

Recovery Insurance

Relapse Prevention

Relapse is one of the biggest fears faced by those beginning a path of recovery. It is scary to think of going back into the chaos of the invader's world after having a taste of freedom. While relapse may be a possibility, it is not inevitable. You have a choice. Breaking free from the prison of your disorder is a choice. It doesn't just happen. And you have the power to make that choice again every day. Hold on to what you have worked for. That House of Being is *yours*. It is up to you what kind of recovery you would like to experience. There is no reason to beat yourself up for having relapse episodes, but you *can* recover without them.

Also, try to remember that a relapse episode does not necessarily reverse all of the re-feeding work you have done. It simply means that you are human. You had a rough day. You tried to go back to a behavior pattern which once seemed to make things better. You saw that it did not work, and you are ready to continue reaching for healthy ways to cope with life's situations. Remember to keep the past in the past. Don't let Guilt and Shame trick you into thinking that you have ruined everything. Just pick up where you left off. Sometimes it takes a few hospitalizations, a long term treatment facility, or years of back-and-forth episodes. It is all okay. There is nothing wrong with you. Work on finding the balance between being gentle with yourself, and being stern enough with yourself to be progressive with your process.

There are ways to help yourself stay on the path of healing, even when temptations arise to revert back to eating disorder behavior. This is a normal part of the recovery process. Be prepared. If you are expecting urges and temptations, they have less of a chance of pulling you back into old behavior patterns. You can learn to see them coming, prepare yourself, and choose to remain centered in your decision to heal.

Know Your Triggers

There are certain people, situations, locations, and interactions which may trigger an urge to re-engage in eating disorder behavior. These triggers are different for everyone. It is helpful to watch for your triggers, and then write them down. This way you will come to know your triggers, and how to avoid them during your vulnerable times. For me, restaurants were a huge trigger. It was too difficult to eat at restaurants for the first few months of recovery. I simply avoided them until I knew I was ready, and then I tried a health food restaurant which felt somewhat safe. Knowing your triggers doesn't mean you have to avoid them always and forever. It may just mean you need a vacation from some people, situations, or locations. I also chose not to see my father for awhile. It wasn't that he did anything wrong. Certain emotions would arise in his presence, and I felt less capable of holding my intention of self-care when I was around him.

Be Selfish!

This is your healing process. It is okay to be somewhat selfish. Do what works for you, regardless of how uncomfortable it may be for others. Warn your loved ones. Let them know that you are going through an intense transformation, and you may not be your "usual self" for awhile. No one else could possibly know what is best for your House of Being. You are learning how to trust your body. Your body is learning how to trust you. You are discovering what it feels like to truly live for perhaps the first time in your life. Many things may change. People may be used to you taking care of everyone, or always agreeing. Those characteristics may be challenged as you come into your power. Keep writing about all of your experiences and changes. In no time you will be a completely different person, ready to share your light with the world.

Remind Yourself "Why"

- Make a list of everything you cannot accomplish until you recover from anorexia/bulimia. What is it keeping you from?

- Make a list of everything your eating disorder has taken from you. What opportunities have passed by because of your disorder?

- Make a list of the negative effects your disorder has had on your life. Has it stolen your joy? Has it altered some relationships?

- Make a "why collage." Cut out some photographs of loved ones, inspirational poetry or slogans, and art or photos symbolizing your goals. Paste them onto a posterboard in a design which feels good to you. Hang your "why collage" somewhere you will see it often. This way, when you start to doubt yourself, you will be reminded of the many reasons for fighting this battle.

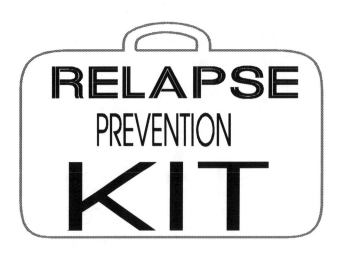

Relapse Prevention Kit

It is time to build your arsenal. The invader will fight back, and you must be prepared. It is best to have some help in place for those moments when the urge to slip back into the garden of weeds seems overwhelming.

You need:

A Relapse Prevention Kit: *A comprehensive help package, complete with tools to distract you, inspire you, remind you, love you, nurture you, guide you, and protect you through a relapse temptation.*

Here are some basic guidelines to help you assemble your relapse prevention kit:

- Your relapse prevention kit should be kept someplace where it is easily accessible. You do not want to have to think about where you put it while you are in the midst of an attack from the invader.

- Choose a suitcase, box, bag, treasure chest, pouch, cabinet, shelf, cubby hole, or backpack for which you have an affinity. You want to use a containment object which you find appealing, or the invader will convince you not to use the kit simply because you do not like the case in which it is kept.

- Decorate the outside of the case. Make it uniquely your own. Glue on some dried flowers and old lace. Cut out photographs of historical warriors and paste them on the outside. Paint it red and put a sign on it that says "USE IN CASE OF EMERGENCY." Make the kit something special, like a healthy friend to support you when times are rough.

- Fill your relapse prevention kit with anything you think may help you in a time of struggle. ANYTHING! Regardless of how silly it may seem. If you have a feeling about any object, include it. Here are some ideas:

    1. Journal and pens or pencils. You may find relief in exposing the thoughts of the invader in writing. Or you could write out all of your fears. Sometimes writing them down makes them appear less overwhelming.

    2. Drawing, art, sketch, or painting supplies. Creativity can relieve stress. Let some toxic emotions out in artistic expression.

    3. A variety of your favorite music. Music can calm your emotions. It may help to lose yourself in your favorite songs for a little while.

    4. A photograph of someone you admire who overcame difficult obstacles in life. Give yourself a good example to remind you of the great accomplishments human beings can achieve.

    5. Photographs of your friends, family, children, or parents. Sometimes it helps to remember that you are not doing this just for you. Other people need you too.

    6. Symbols to represent your future goals. For example, if you are planning to take a trip to Alaska, include a brochure about that state and a list of all the things you would like to do there. This will remind you that staying in or returning to your disorder means forfeiting your future.

    7. On a day when you are feeling especially strong, write a letter to yourself. In it, tell yourself all the reasons why you are glad you chose to recover. Tell yourself, "I am proud of you!" and "I believe in you!" Tell yourself that you know you can do it! Put this letter in your kit. When you read it, it will remind you of how good you felt, and that you can feel that good again. If you climbed out of a hole once, you must be able to climb out again. And this time you just might climb a little further.

    8. A comforting childhood keepsake. A tattered old teddy bear, your favorite bed time story, the blanket you used to sleep with. These may provide some nurturing for the scared little child inside of you.

    9. Safe foods. If you are being restrictive, choose some "safe foods" you know you will eat. This way, you can at least eat something, even if it isn't your complete meal plan. Perhaps it will bridge the gap, and make it easier to eat next time.

    10. A list of friends to call. List the names and phone numbers of anyone who may be able to talk you through a tough spot. Choose a variety of people. Good listeners, logical people, friends who make you laugh, friends who will come over or let you come over if it would help. Be honest with them. Say, "I am calling you instead of purging," or, "I am calling you instead of restricting," or, "I am having a hard day. Could we just talk for a while?"

11. Your therapist's telephone number. If you feel you need some professional help, it would be nice to have the number readily available.
12. Your favorite funny movie or a joke book. Distract yourself with laughter. Laughter is good for energy, and it releases stress.
13. Your "emergency gear." Buy a toy siren, a flag, flashing lights, an emergency outfit with reflectors (like fireman's gear), a walkie-talkie, and flares. Have a genuine emergency! Do it BIG! Turn on the siren, flash the lights, run around the neighborhood (or your house), wave the flag, call out a distress signal. You will have so much fun producing your emergency, you will forget about your relapse urge. This fun exercise will lighten the whole thing up. It will show how ridiculous the invader really is, and how powerful you really are.

The most important thing to remember about relapse is that you have a choice. You don't have to relapse, and if you do, you do not have to stay there. Sometimes it takes a few attempts to climb those clouds. You may have to test out some equipment, or have the right climb team. Try different things until you reach that perfect combination. You don't have to climb perfectly, but you do have to climb.

<u>SELF-CHECK</u>

Shade in what portion of your being is still controlled by the eating disorder.

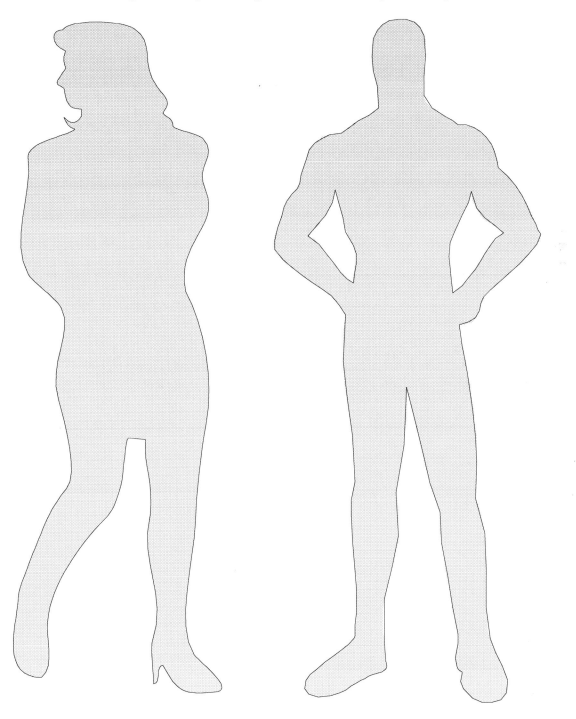

CHAPTER TEN

? *Frequently Asked Questions* ?

During the time I facilitated a support group I took note of some commonly asked questions. While each experience of an eating disorder is unique, together they share some common characteristics. Therefore, some similar concerns and questions arise among those being affected by anorexia and bulimia. Also, a sense of hope can be gained from learning how someone else pushed through some of the same obstacles along the path to healing. Reading the questions asked by others may help you feel less alone during your process, whether you are the person with the eating disorder, a friend, a spouse, or a family member.

Q. **Do you know when your eating disorder started?**

It is difficult to identify the exact point at which my eating disorder began. The appearance of eating disorder behavior, and the appearance of the invader, are two very different things. I lived inside the belief that something was wrong with me long before I began restricting or purging. I remember as early as kindergarten worrying about what others were thinking about me. I don't know what planted the infected seed. Perhaps it was one, distinct event which occurred as early as infancy. Perhaps it was simply a progression of impressions made upon my pure spirit, which accumulated into low self-esteem. I think we can all look at our lives and remember many instances which could have contributed to an idea that something was wrong with us. Receiving a dirty look from someone in class. Being shunned by peers. Making mistakes. Being rejected. Telling lies. Not receiving adequate love and affection during childhood. In every situation the message was the same: "There is something wrong with you!" I think it is helpful to step out of identifying specific occurrences, and go after the underlying source of it all. My invader was taking up so much space in my life, it eventually surfaced in the form of an eating disorder, and could no longer be ignored. I do not know why my invader showed up as anorexia/bulimia instead of some other unhealthy coping mechanism.

I do believe that people with eating disorders have been chosen for some intense self-work. One cannot live without food. Food is everywhere. This disorder is a constant state. It is a huge obstacle. It distracts one from everything else. And if it is not identified, extracted, and transformed, it is fatal. I believe that recovering from an eating disorder is a great method for developing unshakable inner strength and confidence. When you defeat the invader, you feel that you can do anything - and you can!

Q. At what point did you know you had an eating disorder?

I was in complete denial until the first time I attended the support group at Beaumont Hospital. Even when I thought I was crazy, and knew something was wrong, I never imagined it was anorexia/bulimia. I did not think I qualified. I thought anorexia/bulimia was a topic on talk shows. I did not think it had anything to do with me. In my mind, I was nowhere near being sick enough to be anorexic/bulimic. Restricting was simply my way of eating healthy. Purging was just my way of dealing with feeling too full. I had myself convinced that I was not doing any damage to my body.

Something deep within me must have known and agreed to attend the support group. Perhaps it was the part of me that noticed I no longer had a choice whether or not to eat. Everything changed when I went to the first meeting. I was listening to other people talk about thoughts that I had been thinking, and habits that I had adopted. It was quite a shock to realize that anorexia/bulimia was exactly what I was dealing with. Part of me wanted to admit it openly so I could escape from its grasp. Another part of me was ashamed. Still another part of me was protective of it, thinking it was all that I had, and all that I was.

Q. What are some of the warning signs that anorexia/bulimia are present?

While every experience of an eating disorder is unique, there are some common symptoms. These could include any or all of the following:

Physical Symptoms:
- weight loss
- fatigue
- cold often
- chest pain
- pale skin
- hair falling out
- layer of fine hair growing on the body
- headaches
- lightheadedness
- dizziness
- passing out
- tooth damage
- digestive disturbances (diarrhea, nausea, acid reflux, hiatal hernia, blood with bowel movement)

Behavioral Symptoms:
- reclusion
- refusal to eat with others
- refusal to eat at social events
- refusal to eat food someone else has prepared
- food restrictions (won't eat after a certain time, won't eat certain foods)
- reading cookbooks
- preparing food for others and not eating
- obsession with appearance
- increase in self-criticism
- loss of interest in usual activities
- excessive talking about food and weight
- frequent weighing
- mood swings
- depression
- exercising more, and at odd times of day or night
- laxative or diuretic use
- use of energy enhancement products (herbal or over the counter)
- inspecting the body in the mirror
- decrease in mental capabilities (forgetful, dropping grades)
- more afraid of gaining weight than anything - even death

Q. What are some of the physical dangers that come with engaging in eating disorder behavior?

Every anorexic/bulimic thinks, "I'm not *that* bad," meaning, "I'm not that sick." Even if you have only purged once, only restricted for one day, only taken diet pills, laxatives, or diuretics once - you ARE that sick. One purge is one too many. Physical repercussions may not even surface until recovery begins. For me, my physical disruptions began after I had made the decision to recover. Every person is different, so the dangers of practicing eating disorder behavior are different for everyone.

Here are some physical repercussions I have seen or heard about:

- kidney dysfunction or failure
- infertility (short or long term)
- ruptured esophagus (which can happen during any purge - the first, twenty-first, or one-hundred and first)
- bone density loss
- joint damage
- heart failure (cardiac arrest)
- muscle atrophy
- loss of brain function
- nerve damage

- anemia
- intestinal/colon damage (especially with laxative use)
- pancreatic damage (long term blood sugar imbalances)
- hair loss
- impaired immune function

Q. **How would you suggest I approach someone who I suspect is suffering from an eating disorder?**

This is a delicate situation. Denial and anger are common reactions to confrontation - especially when someone is trying to hide the truth. When the invader suspects that someone is coming close to exposing it, the guards are sent out. These guards lie, have a temper tantrum, or whatever else will make that person sorry for prying into the invader's territory. The invader will fight for what it has over-taken. This is why paranoia is common with eating disorders. Every anorexic is sure that there is a secret conspiracy to make her gain weight. Most will not eat food anyone else has prepared. Most will not eat in front of other people. This paranoia is simply the invader guarding its prisoner.

The idea must be to sneak around the invader while it is asleep, and try to talk to the part of that person which is not completely under the invader's control. This is not easy. Timing and sincerity are very important. My mother happened to wait to approach me until I was miserable and afraid, and knew something was wrong. So I was somewhat receptive. While I had no intention of gaining weight or putting a stop to my dieting, I had reached a miserable state, and I wanted help. Also, my mother did not attack me or accuse me; she asked me. She asked me if I had been losing weight, and how much more I wanted to lose. She was sincerely inquiring about what I had been doing, so I did not feel the need to be defensive.

I believe that everyone who is suffering from anorexia and bulimia wants help, but the invader does everything it can to block that intention. That person who is being held prisoner must realize she is in prison, and that she no longer wants to be there. Only then can any kind of help penetrate the layer of invader-mind which is controlling her world.

I suggest giving the person a self-test (see below). Don't ask to see the results. Just let the person do the test in private. My sister gave me a self-test before I admitted I had anorexia/bulimia. I filled it out by myself. After I read my results, something in me admitted that I did have an eating disorder. Even if no one else ever saw that test, and even if I lied in my answers, a seed was planted. Something changed. Giving the self-test is a gentle way to begin "the conversation." "The conversation" can last minutes, hours, days, weeks, months, or years. The amount of time it takes for someone to accept help varies depending on how long the invader has been present, which phase of the disorder the person is in, and many other factors.

It is difficult to say what approach is best. Regardless of the technique used, always speak and listen from your heart. Perhaps you can tap into the part of that person who is lost, afraid, and imprisoned by the invader.

Self-Test

Circle true or false.

~ I cannot eat a meal without worrying about its calorie or fat content.
> True
> False

~ I lie about what I eat.
> True
> False

~ I hide food and eat when no one else is around.
> True
> False

~ I engage in purging behavior (induced vomiting, laxative use, diuretic use, over exercising).
> True
> False

~ I restrict my intake of food.
> True
> False

~ I am only happy when I am not eating, or I am not near food.
> True
> False

~ I avoid social functions when there is food involved.
> True
> False

~ I cannot remember the last time I ate without worrying about gaining weight.
> True
> False

~ I weight myself at least once a day.
> True
> False

~ I have trouble concentrating because of fatigue, or distracting thoughts about food.
> True
> False

~ Even when I lose weight, I think I need to lose more.
> True
> False

~ I would rather die than gain weight.
> True
> False

Did you answer true to any of the above questions? If you did, this is a sign that you could have an eating disorder. Each true answer is a reason to seek help. Talk to someone - your family, your counselor, your doctor, your friends.

Q. **How did you handle the guilt which arose from knowing that you "did this to yourself?"**

One of the hardest things to overcome is guilt. I remember looking at the mess my life had become and thinking, "I can't believe I did this to myself." It was so overwhelming that it came close to causing a relapse several times. It was difficult to face the fact that everything that was happening was a result of decisions I had made.

The way I had to process this guilt was to realize that feeling guilty about it would only hold me in the invader's grasp. I talked to my mom about it, and she made it clear that she did not want me to feel guilty about all that had happened. She only wanted me to be well and happy.

Another thing which helped me deal with guilt was the realization that everything happens for a reason. Every moment of my life has led me to this moment. I had to look deeper into my eating disorder. I found that if I would not have experienced such a trauma, I would not be as strong as I am. If I had never come so close to death, I would not cherish every moment of life the way I do. If the invader had never grown big enough to surface in my life, I might still be under its control. I "did this to myself". It was a part of my story, and it gave me the opportunity to change the ending.

Q. **Do you believe it is possible to recover completely?**

Yes!

Q. **How did you overcome the fear of food?**

I took my power back from the fear monster's grasp. It was slow and gradual. Not every battle was easy. Not every battle ended in victory. But eventually, I was able to see that if I did not overcome this fear of food, I would never be able to live the life I wanted to live. The world of fear became too small for me to live in. I decided I wanted more than what the limited world of anorexia/bulimia could offer me.

- I said affirmations.
- I journaled or talked about every fear that came up, so it would be exposed and lose power over my behavior.
- I knew I had to gain weight in order to be healthy and happy, so I decided to try to relax about the food at least until my weight stabilized. And by the time I reached a safe weight, I was not afraid anymore. I felt better, and I saw the difference between living in anorexia/bulimia, and living in freedom and activity.
- I looked at my goal, and decided that accepting food as my ally was the only way to reach that goal.
- I kept my eye on the prize. I wanted my life back. I could either stay alive and push through the fear, or I could give in to the fear and die. I finally saw that it was my choice. I could change my mind.

- I stuck with my decision. I promised myself I would re-feed, and I actively pursued that goal.

Consistency is the key. The more you do exactly what you are afraid of, the less you are afraid. The unfamiliar becomes the familiar, and what made you afraid, now makes you strong.

Q. How long does it take for the negative inner voices to go away?

The disappearance of negative self-talk is gradual. When you actively participate in your healing process (eat, say affirmations, journal, etc.) you are feeding the part of you which wants to live. As you feed that part, it gradually becomes stronger and takes up more space in your mind. As the healthy part of you grows, there is less room for the invader, and the toxic messages begin to fade away. It doesn't happen all at once. Some days the toxic voices are more prominent than others. It is like cleaning out a room in your house. As you organize the space, and throw away what is no longer useful, there is more room for new plants, furniture, rugs, etc.

Remember, the invader will fight for its existence within you. It may become more difficult before it becomes easier. This is normal. Keep being active in your recovery process. Let the invader know that you are serious about living. Soon it will move on to an easier target.

Here are some tools I used to conquer negative self-talk:

- Expose the lies! Talk about the toxic messages that are running through your mind. The more you expose them, the less power they have over you.
- Scare them away. Yell out loud, "Stop! You are lying! That is weed food, and I am a flower!"
- Practice positive self-talk. Do the affirmations, be gentle to yourself.
- Hang affirmation signs all over the house.
- Go to support groups and share about your toxic inner messages. It helps to know that other people are facing the same challenges.

Q. What will I do with my time instead of obsessing over my food rituals?

As you make room in your life you will be amazed at the wonderful opportunities which arise. You will have more energy, so you will want to do more. If anything, you will find yourself trying to do *too* much. I remember finding myself wondering why I had wasted so much time worrying about food and weight. As you stop giving so much time and energy to dying, you have more energy to channel into living!

Q. What made you ask for help?

There were many factors.

First, I remember thinking I was insane. I could not concentrate. I thought about food constantly. I went to health food stores, walked around and read food labels; and left without buying anything. I read cookbooks in my spare time. Every moment of every day was consumed with food thoughts. I had no other interests. I thought I was going to have to be admitted into a mental hospital. Something inside me knew that life was not supposed to be that way.

Second, I realized that I no longer had a choice whether to eat or not eat. Even if I wanted to eat, I couldn't. Something inside me, some powerful shadow-self, had imprisoned my ability to choose, and I could not seem to take it back.

The third factor surfaced when my mother asked me how much more weight I wanted to lose. My immediate response was, "Just five more pounds." As I said that sentence, I realized that was what I had been saying for the previous forty pounds of weight loss. In that moment I saw that whatever was going on inside me really had nothing to do with how much I weighed. It would never be enough. I saw that I was on a dead end road.

Most importantly, I reached a point where I knew that whatever happened after asking for help had to be better than the way I was living.

Q. How did you deal with having to gain weight?

Gaining weight is a horrifying idea to anyone facing re-feeding. But this is the invader's perspective. The invader has tricked us into mislabeling food - and pounds. It is time to adopt a new idea of gaining weight. It will save your life, it will free you from the invader, and it will allow you to reach your dreams.

I think we all play a game at the beginning of recovery. We pretend we can recover without actually gaining any weight. The disorder will not allow us to see how illogical and impossible this idea is. This is why the games of not adding fat, or exercising more are so common during the first stages of re-feeding. Not every recovery is the same, but there are some basic rules.

- You have to gain weight.
- You have to stop purging.
- You have to stop taking laxatives and diuretics.
- You have to eat.

I tried escaping every one of these rules at some point during the first stages of re-feeding. Soon I saw that escaping recovery meant destroying my life. When you reach a point at which the disorder has ruined every part of your life, the only choice left is to push through the fear, and gain the weight.

Here are some things I did which made it a bit easier.

- I threw away the scale. I stopped weighing myself. I decided not to give my energy to numbers on a machine.
- I stopped talking about weight in general. I wanted to concentrate on other things.
- I threw away all of my "sick clothes." I canceled out the notion that someday I would be able to fit into the small sizes again.

- I did a journal exercise describing what I wanted to be remembered for, and found that it was not for my physical appearance.
- I stopped watching television and reading magazines. I found that when I "unplugged," I did not compare myself to others as much.
- I talked about the discomfort of gaining weight. I talked about my fears. I shared my inner world so that I did not feel alone.
- I looked at people I thought were beautiful, and realized that none of them were underweight. In fact, most of them were slightly "overweight." I began to reform my ideas of beauty. I realized that I did not have to think how the media thought, or how anyone else thought. I could decide what I thought was beautiful.
- I decided to become a woman instead of a remaining a little girl. I realized I loved women's bodies. I loved hips and bellies. I was born to be a woman, and that was what I wanted to be. I decided to embrace my own true nature.
- I wrote a lot in my journal. I joyously documented the good days, and unloaded my fear thoughts on challenging days. Through writing, I learned to clearly express my emotions, and become my own friend - through thick and thin.
- I made gaining weight my project. My life revolved around it for a while. I needed to give my body that attention and affection. The body is neglected during an eating disorder. It needs love in order to blossom.
- I realized that I wanted to be happy. The invader tricked me into thinking I would be happy if I lost weight, but I was miserable! I faced the fact that anorexia/bulimia did not work. It made everything worse.

After a while, eating became easier. As I became healthier, I could see that it was taking a long time to gain weight. I saw that I would have to eat a lot of food in order to reach my goal weight. At that point I decided to have fun with it. I thought I might as well enjoy what I was eating since I had to gain the weight anyway. I began experimenting a lot with vegetarian cookbooks. Food actually became fun again.

I found that the more consistent I was with re-feeding, the better I felt. As I gained weight, I gradually came to accept my body as it was, instead of trying to change it. The healing process happens perfectly when you do your part. If you keep eating, each day you will find yourself feeling stronger and more alert. You are bringing yourself back to life.

Q. What was the turning point in your recovery?

It is difficult to identify the exact turning point. There were several important incidents which brought me closer to letting go of the invader.

One day I was at work (I was an assistant manager of a clothing store). A friend of mine, whom I had not seen in a long time, came in to see me. He asked me what I had been doing, and I realized that all I had been doing was losing weight. I had nothing else to talk about. I felt insignificant. My life had no meaning. When this happened, I saw how I had been giving my life away to a disease, instead of living.

Telling people about my situation also played an important role. When I exposed the invader by telling people that I was trying to gain weight, the responses I received surprised me. Every co-worker, friend, and relative had been concerned about me. They were all relieved to hear that the problem was being addressed, and they had been afraid to approach me about my appearance, as well as about my obvious personality changes. Their concern and awareness made me see how silly anorexia and bulimia were. I was not fooling anyone but myself. They all knew it wasn't going to work, it just took me awhile to realize it. The support I received made a huge difference in how my recovery progressed. It helped me build a life to live into, so I could leave the dead world of the invader behind.

The physical complications which arose also served as motivation. Seeing all the damage I had done to my body, and how close I had come to not being alive anymore, ignited something inside of me that was ready to fight. As soon as I couldn't walk, I saw what a miracle it was to be able to walk. More and more I realized what an absolute privilege it was to be alive, and to have a body. I felt humble, and ready to care for the gift of life which so generously had been given to me.

Q. How did your family help you during your recovery?

My family helped me in more ways than I could ever list in this book! Here are just a few:

- They made sure I knew I was loved, no matter what.
- They learned about anorexia and bulimia by reading books and going to support group meetings.
- They asked me what it was like *for me*. They let me talk, without correcting me or criticizing me. They listened to what was going on inside of my head, and tried to understand what seemed so foreign to them.
- They kept themselves healthy and strong.
- They tolerated my many moods (which were quite difficult at times). They let me cry when I needed to cry, and laughed with me when I was ready to laugh.
- They reminded me of my own greatness when I could not see it.
- They told me the truth. When I was sick, no one pretended not to notice. They told me when they were scared. They told me when I did not look healthy. They told me when they did not understand. We talked with each other.
- They created a safe and supportive environment in which to heal. They let my health be important. They let it be okay for me to need their help, while making it clear that I needed to do the work.
- They prayed for me, and with me.
- They believed that I could do it.

Q. How long does it take to feel normal?

What is normal? "Normal" is different for every person. At the beginning of my recovery process, I had the idea that I was working toward being normal again. I thought that after doing a certain amount of work, I would reach a place in my life where the change would stop, and my world would be predictable and manageable. I thought it would be enough of a gift to be able to eat food when I was hungry, without having to endure endless self-torture. I thought I would settle into a rhythm, and just live out my days, happy and recovered. For some people, this point is as far as they want to go, and that is fine. After a certain amount of time (which is different for everyone) you will find yourself at peace with food, feeling healthy and strong, and actively participating in life. You will find yourself gradually experiencing less challenging days. Slowly, the inner voices will quiet down. You will again want to be social. You will have ambition. You will feel "normal."

This is a wonderful place to reach. You believe that you can do anything. You refused to let the invader continue to run your life. And you can take it a step further. This process has given you great gifts of endurance, perseverance, and strength. I believe that those of us who reach this point can take those gifts and do something to make the world a better place. We are special. We have overcome a battle, and reclaimed our lives from the invader. We all have the power to apply our abilities. You must decide what that means for you. For me, part of it was writing this book. I knew that if I was given enough strength to endure the battle I fought against anorexia/bulimia, there was a special purpose for me on planet Earth.

What is your purpose? Do you want to be "normal," or do you want to strive to be extraordinary? It's up to you where you want to go from here.

CHAPTER ELEVEN

*Tips For Family
and
Friends*

Watching a loved one struggle through anorexia or bulimia can be terrifying. You don't know what to say, what not to say, how to help, what to do, or if they will survive. It is a confusing time. It is normal to feel helpless and distraught.

Eating disorder behavior is not easily understood by someone who has never traveled that road. It seems irrational, destructive, and incomprehensible. Your loved one exists within a world you have never seen. She is hearing and speaking a language which was developed by the invader. She is seeing through eyes which are glazed over by fear. She is living beneath a thick cloud of self-doubt, self-destruction, and deep confusion.

There is no way to determine what exactly will penetrate that world and begin to alter the perception of life. Reaching your loved one often requires diligence and creativity, and it always requires unconditional, continuous love.

Here are some suggestions for how to make it through this challenging process:

Take Care of You

One of the most important and most difficult things to remember is to take care of yourself. This does not mean that you cannot be supportive, or that you cannot help your loved one. It means that the first thing you must do is take care of you. By keeping yourself strong, healthy, and calm, you can serve as a powerful example of self-care, self-esteem, and self-respect. This is what a person who is trying to recover needs more than anything. Your loved one needs to see that it is safe and desirable to live without dysfunction.

Here are some ideas of how to take care of yourself:

- Keep eating in a healthy way.
- Maintain your spiritual support.
- Get enough rest.
- Take bubble baths.
- Spend time in nature.
- Do what makes you happy. Don't give up your own important activities (classes, hobbies, exercise routines).

When a loved one is ill, it is easy to drop your life and just take care of that person. However, this does not serve everyone involved. The person who is recovering must do the work. That person has attracted this situation in order to learn some valuable lessons. By all means be available and supportive, but not at the expense of your own well being. When you are feeling tired or drained, step back and do something for yourself. Practice some self-care. The healthier you are, the more you will be able to offer appropriate support.

Affection and Attention

Healing touch is extremely important for everyone, especially those who are involved in a recovery process. People recovering from eating disorders have withdrawn and withheld love from their physical bodies. To them, the body is an alien, an enemy, or a project. They may think of the body as disgusting, unlovable, and grotesque. The body is starving for affection and attention. Often people recovering will not request, and may even avoid, healing touch. The invader has convinced them that they are not deserving of affection and attention. The invader convinces them to shy away from exactly what is needed to enhance the healing process. You can help to change all of this by offering some healthy affection and attention.

Here are some ideas:
- Hug more often.
- Sit closer on the couch.
- Hold hands while talking.
- Offer a hand or foot massage.
- Brush or style hair.
- Give a manicure.
- Dance together.

The body does not communicate with words, it communicates with touch. Giving some affection and attention will send the healthy message to the body that it deserves to be cared for, and that there is nothing wrong with it. Also, any type of physical attention and affection, like massage, will increase the overall energy flow in the body, which will make the healing process more efficient and holistic. Affection and attention help the body wake up and begin rebuilding what has been lost through the abuse that comes with anorexia/bulimia.

Learn About Their World

People with anorexia/bulimia live in a completely different world. They think differently, listen differently, speak differently, and feel differently. Everyone they see is potentially someone who will try to make them "fat." While they are appearing to communicate with you, the invader is constantly whispering or screaming inside of their heads, telling them that you are a liar, and that you want to make them gain weight. It is difficult to break through that layer of "invader-talk." The first step is recognizing that they live in a different world, and attempting

130

to learn about that world. Learning about the world in which your loved one is living will bring a deeper understanding.

Here are some things you can do:

• Ask your loved what it is like to live with the invader.

• Make it clear that you want to understand - become the student.

• Read books about anorexia/bulimia.

• Attend support group meetings.

• Talk to other parents, siblings, and spouses.

While you can never know exactly what an eating disorder feels like, becoming educated about the world of eating disorders can help you gain a deeper understanding, which will allow you and your loved one to feel closer in this challenging time.

Toxic Messages

As we watch our loved ones struggle with body image, we begin to notice how saturated society is with toxic messages about self-image. Everywhere we turn there are advertisements for diet pills or weight loss schemes. Every commercial is telling you there is something wrong with you, and the product they are selling will fix it. Unfortunately, it is much more common for people to complain or insult their bodies than it is for people to accept and love their bodies. This is unnatural. You must stop these toxic messages from programming your family. And if they already have, it is time to change!

Here are some ways you can become an example of a healthy self-image for your loved one:

• Stop criticizing your own body.

• Stop criticizing the appearance of others.

• Stop talking about bodies in general, placing more importance on heart and soul.

• Don't watch commercials and stop buying magazines.

• Stop dieting.

• Don't use favorite food items as a reward item for achievements. This will help prevent the replacement of healthy emotional processing with physical food. Let the feeling of achievement itself be the reward! Allow that emotional high to be felt, instead of halting it by stimulating the body.

Always Tell the Truth

It is imperative to always be truthful with your loved one. Lying is an unhealthy coping skill that often accompanies eating disorders. You can demonstrate *healthy* coping skills. You can show that telling the truth always brings more valuable results. If your loved one asks you a question, tell the truth - even when it would be easier to lie. Show her that you will push through the difficulty together. The questions may be uncomfortable, covering topics such as death, spirituality, self-esteem, weight gain or loss, and repressed childhood memories.

Speak and listen from your heart. When you are afraid, say so. Tell her you love her. Be honest and open with your feelings. This will give her the permission to do the same with you.

If you do not know the answer to a question, suggest researching the topic together. Perhaps a doctor, counselor, friend, or publication would be able to help. The questions which surface for those recovering are very important. Eating disorders can cause many intense psychological and emotional symbols to surface.

Life can seem difficult and overwhelming. The invader will try to convince us that it is easier to lie than to resolve issues. Telling the truth is one way to face uncomfortable situations, reclaim your energy from the fear monster, and strengthen relationships.

Listen

The best way to understand a person who is facing an eating disorder is to listen. Listen without interrupting, without criticizing, and without correcting. Let your loved one talk, cry, and wonder; and just be there, quiet and stable. Attempt listening in silence, only speaking if a question is asked. If there is an uncomfortable silence, encourage your loved one to continue sharing. You could say something like, "I appreciate you sharing with me, please continue," or, "Thank you for telling me how you are feeling, it helps me to understand."

Listening sincerely is one way to reinforce self-worth. You don't always have to completely understand everything being said. Your presence is what matters. People will often begin to figure out their own answers once they open and share.

Encourage Exposure

Give permission. Allow any moods which arise. Let confusion, anger, and sadness be okay. The only way to push through a toxic emotional state is to fully express it, and find what is on the other side. As toxic emotions are purged, they have less power. It may be that your loved one will experience depression. Instead of trying to "cheer her up," try to help her reach the cause of the depression. Encourage her to talk or journal about how she feels. There is much to be learned from inner sadness.

Let your loved one be. Don't try to make her into what you want her to be. Don't ask, "Where is the old Cathy I used to know?" More than likely it is best to let go of that "old Cathy." That "old Cathy" is part of the old patterns which brought her to self-destruction. Something new must be constructed. The old ways don't work. The goal of recovery cannot be to "get back to normal." It must be to spread your wings and fly! Fulfill your potential! Spread out and experience your inherent greatness!

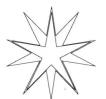

Pray

Prayer changes everything. It connects us to possibilities we cannot imagine ourselves. It reminds us that we are not in charge, and that we are safe in the hands of God. We don't always know what to do next, so we must turn to the only One who could know. Regardless of what entity you recognize, or what religion you practice, prayer can bring a peace of mind which can be found no other way.

There is no wrong way to pray. Simply be sincere. Pray as if you are talking to your best friend. Pray in song. Cry in your prayer, surrendering all of your pain and confusion. Pray by picturing everyone you know surrounded by healing white light. Pray together with your loved one, asking for the strength to push through this challenge, and the wisdom to see

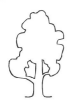

the lessons in it. Pray in a traditional way, or in a new way. Pray in silence, or out loud. Write a letter to God. Try to see God in everything - even suffering. Especially suffering! Go outside and find your favorite tree. Find God in that tree. Talk to that tree about all of your troubles. Be creative. Pray a different way every day if that works for you.

Healthy Communication

Communication is one of the greatest challenges we face, especially during the challenge of an eating disorder. It can seem as though an understanding will never be reached. There are some simple communication tools which, when implemented, can lead to satisfying communication interactions.

One of these tools is the use of "I" and "you" messages. These messages allow each person to talk about how he/she is feeling, and to take responsibility for those feelings. An "I" message is used when you are talking about your needs/desires. It describes how you are feeling, and what needs of yours are not being met. Examples of appropriate "I" messages are, "I feel misunderstood," or, "I feel underestimated," or, "I feel afraid." "I" messages also speak about needs, "I need a hug," "I need you to listen," "I don't want to talk." These are examples of "I" messages. The focus is on the needs and feelings of the speaker. "I" messages do not blame, and do not accuse. If possible, the word "you" should be left out altogether.

"You" messages are used when you are trying to understand the other person's feelings, needs, and desires. It begins with the idea that you do not know, and that you are trying to learn. If you cannot bring this attitude, do not even try a "you" message - it will come out wrong.

"You" messages are not used to lay blame, or to make people wrong. They are a reflective tool. "You" messages are used in response to "I" messages, as an attempt to clearly hear and understand what the other person is expressing. Some appropriate "you" messages are, " Oh, so you are feeling misunderstood and underestimated? I can hear that." "You sound angry." "You want to be left alone." "It sounds to me like what you are saying is that you need your privacy." It is important to keep "you" messages tentative. We are asking not because we think we know, but because we are trying to understand. If we ask tentatively we give the other person a chance to correct, and tell us how he/she is really feeling.

Everything changes when people feel heard. There is no longer any need to argue. Try implementing "I" and "you" messages during a conversation. If you notice you have gone back to old ways of communicating, stop, and begin "I" and "you" messages again. It takes a while to learn, but the results are phenomenal.

Another simple tool which can increase the accuracy of what is heard and said is the use of breath. While in conversation, take a deep breath before responding to anything anyone says. This will calm the mind, and possibly help you stay out of defense mechanisms or argumentation.

If communication is unbearable, contact a qualified mediator. Having a third party present can sometimes effectively bridge the gap of understanding.

Encourage Separation From the Invader

When you suspect that your loved one is in the grasp of the invader, Shame, Guilt, or the fear monster, gently ask, "Who said that? You, or the invader?" Help them see that they are not the disorder. Help them separate from the thoughts of the invader. Ask for a description of the invader. Ask what it looks like, what it sounds like, what it says. Ask about the fear monster. What does it look like? What does it try to make you afraid of? You could say something like, " Is that invader trying to convince you that something is wrong with you? Because there is nothing wrong with you!"

Fight the Invader as a Team

This is an opportunity to work on your own invader. We all have one! Whether it surfaces as an eating disorder, or some other form of unhealthy coping. It may be easier to fight the invader as a team.

Here are some activities you could do together:

• Sit down face to face with your loved one, and take turns saying, "There is nothing wrong with you." It will feel strange at first. Either of you may giggle, cry, or fidget. Say it over and over to each other until all of the discomfort disappears. The discomfort is the resistance of the invader. When the discomfort is gone, you have broken the barrier, and you may be able to hear each other.

• Make signs together that say, "No invader allowed!" or, "I don't believe you, invader!" and tape them up around the house.

• Play a game and pretend you are playing against the invader.

• Choose a breakable object to represent the invader. Go outside to a safe place, and smash it with a bat.

Exposing and defeating the invader as a team will provide motivation that can be found no other way. Your loved one will feel less alone, and more capable of reaching the goal of self-care.

Look At the Big Picture

It can be easy to become caught up in the struggle of anorexia/bulimia. It can seem like a tragedy. When you feel overwhelmed by the circumstances of this challenge, try to step back, and remember that life's challenges are life's greatest gifts. We would never learn anything if we never struggled. We would never grow if we were never pulled out of our comfort zone. Think about what valuable lessons you are learning from this experience - lessons that could not be learned any other way. Perhaps this is bringing you closer to your loved one. Perhaps this is causing you to reevaluate your priorities. Perhaps this is igniting your spiritual life. Write and talk about what you are learning. Trust that there is a larger meaning to all that is happening. Look at the big picture. This is an opportunity to change and grow, and to reform your life based on new goals and ideals.

CHAPTER TWELVE

Cloud Climbing

It Is Time!

Clearing the invader out of your life is not easy work. It takes dedication and courage. It takes consistency and diligence. Healing will consume every moment of every day. What could be more important? If you procrastinate about healing, you will simply remain dead. It is time! IT IS TIME! Time to embrace healing. Time to embrace life. Time to stop being afraid.

You must climb those clouds. They do not clear on their own. You must intentionally overcome that which holds you back from reaching the break in the clouds. You must fight your way to the top of that cloud mountain, refusing to be stopped by anything. You must blaze your own trail, and sing your own song along the way. Use the tools which work for you. Find your motivation, and do not forget it. You must make *your* quest and claim *your* prize.

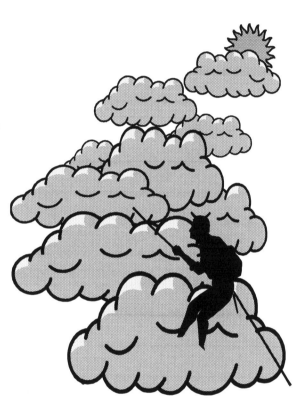

Saying good-bye to the invader is scary. You are letting go of the mask with which you identified yourself. You are going into unfamiliar territory. But you have a choice in perspective, which changes everything. You can choose to see this struggle of recovery as an unfortunate burden to bear, or you can choose to see it as an exciting adventure; a colorful twist of fate; a precious second chance at life.

It is time to say good-bye to the cloak which has hidden your true self for too long. It is time to see what is under there, waiting to blossom. It is time to let yourself be the flower you are - the person you are meant to become during your life. It is time to reach for something bigger, something more meaningful. The world of anorexia/bulimia is too small for you to live in. If you stay there, you will remain dead to all the life you could have lived. You must choose to break out of the tomb of the invader, and find a world more conducive to your inherent greatness; a world in which you can shine!

JOURNAL BREAK: Saying Good-bye

Saying good-bye to that imposter is not easy, but it is the key to finding a break in the clouds. Write a letter to your eating disorder. Thank it for doing its best to help you cope with life, and let it know that you are going to take it from here. Some partnerships are good for awhile, but become toxic and dangerous. There are some things you must outgrow along your life path. Let it know that you have work to do on this planet; a purpose to fulfill, and it cannot accompany you where you need to go.

Even though it may be difficult to see now, someday you will look back on your eating disorder as a great teacher. Among many other great lessons, eating disorders, in retrospect, instill a profound gratitude for the gift of life we have been given.

Dear Eating Disorder:

Breaking Free From Prison

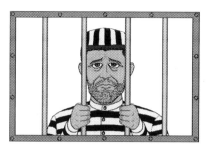

By climbing the clouds, you are breaking out of the "there is something wrong with you" prison. You are escaping from a dingey cell in the invader's dungeon. You are leaving the guards (Guilt and Shame) and the warden (Fear Monster) behind. You are going to climb the wall of self-doubt, and claim the freedom which is rightfully yours. You can never give up. If you do, you will be accepting the dull, limited, and mechanical life of a prisoner. You are innocent, and were wrongly imprisoned. It is time to break out! Fight for your freedom. Fight for your life!

JOURNAL BREAK: The Prison

Write or illustrate a story of your prison break. Be specific. Describe your cell, the other inmates, the warden and guards. Draw a map of the prison. Describe the escape route you chose. What obstacles and dangers did you dodge on your way out? Tell the entire story of your escape. Where do you want to go once you are free? Do you know any other people who have escaped?

Trusting Those Who Have Gone Before

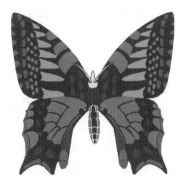

While immersed in the world of anorexia/bulimia, it is difficult to imagine what it would be like to eat without worry, and feel happy regardless of your weight. This is where trust comes in. A leap of faith is necessary. You must place your belief in those who have gone before you, those who have broken free from prison. This is why support groups are so helpful. Often there are people experiencing different stages of recovery, which allows you to watch the process before you go through it. You have to trust that it does become easier, and the clouds do clear. A caterpillar in a cocoon cannot imagine how it feels to be a butterfly until it becomes that butterfly. You are in the process of breaking open your cocoon so that you can fly. Trust the other butterflies. They are proof that you can do it!

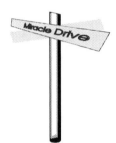

Live On Miracle Drive

Try seeing everything as a miracle - because everything IS a miracle! The air you breathe, the body you inhabit, the earth you live on, the emotions you feel. Your heart beats continuously without being plugged in. Your brain thinks thoughts and formulates sentences. Your eyes allow you to see things. Your heart can feel love. You can laugh. Live inside of the idea that you are a miracle. Everything you see is a miracle. Everyone you know is a miracle. Don't take it for granted that you exist. Live on Miracle Drive. Reside there. Pack up and move away from Stress Street, Worry Way, and Low Self-Esteem Boulevard. You have the choice, you have some tools. It is time to act. It is time to move. Leave the slums of self-abuse behind you, and choose the serene neighborhood of self-care.

JOURNAL BREAK: Your Miracle Drive

Imagine a perfect neighborhood. A quiet street with tall trees and nice homes. Perhaps children are playing outside on the front lawns. Perhaps there is a park nearby. Perhaps your perfect neighborhood is in a rural setting, with a farm and some animals. Whatever seems perfect to you, start spending time there. Write a story with your perfect neighborhood and your house on Miracle Drive as the setting. Perhaps there could be a correlation between your house on Miracle Drive and your House of Being? When you feel stress, close your eyes and picture yourself in your house in your perfect neighborhood. This could be a meditation tool which could be useful in calming your thoughts. If writing is helpful to you, purchase a journal specifically for this Miracle Drive project. Write about Miracle Drive every day.

Next, you could try to walk on Miracle Drive all the time. In your journal, take notes about all of the miracles in your life. What miracles are you noticing that you have never noticed before? Gradually, you will begin to see that everything is a miracle, and that everything is perfect when you choose to live on Miracle Drive.

> *"We usually take the material world with all its wonders and complexities for granted and reject the possibility that there might be other domains of reality. However, if we think about it, the sheer mystery of existence - the fact that anything exists at all, and that it is possible to experience worlds of any kind - is so stupendous and overwhelming that it makes the question about the specifics of their nature and content a trivial one."*
>
> *- Stanislov Grof*
> *The Cosmic Game*

Gratitude

> *"The gods visit us through illness."*
> **-Carl Jung**

There is so much to be thankful for. Your family, your home, your eyes, your brain, your dog, your friends, your existence! Start a gratitude journal! Every day write down something for which you are grateful. This activity reminds us not to take all of the "little" gifts for granted.   After a while, you may just find yourself being thankful for life's challenges. Your greatest qualities have probably been a product of your most difficult experiences. Live in gratitude, and there will never be any reason to be anything less than delighted with life.

Write Your Story

If you were to write out what has happened in your life up to this point, you would have quite an interesting story. You live your story. You speak, whisper, cry, and scream your lines. You wear your different costumes. You walk into and out of various plots with many different characters. Life is a story. We live the story as we live our lives. Most often, however, we forget that we can also *write* the story. We can decide on our lines, choose our costumes, create our plots, and select a cast of characters. **Who wrote the story you have been living so far?** Have you been settling for what other people have written for you? Have you been playing a part which is not your own?

JOURNAL BREAK: A New Chapter

You have a choice! It is time to start a new chapter. Who do you want in your story? What part do you want to play? What events are you going to write about? How are you going to show up in your life? Write it down. Write your story. This is a brand new chapter, ready to be filled with your recovery, your health, and your power!

PEACE TREATY

I,_____, agree to a complete armistice with the invader. I acknowledge that the invader has been a teacher to me, and that it is time for us to part ways peacefully.

I do not blame the invader for the struggle I have endured, rather I thank the invader for the valuable lessons I have learned from experiencing such challenges.

In setting each other free, the invader and I may both become what we are meant to become.

I am ready to move on from the invader's garden of weeds, into the "there is nothing wrong with me" garden of flowers.

I am willing to use the healthy coping skills I am learning instead of relying on the invader's services. I bid the invader a sincere farewell, for I no longer need to hurt myself in order to learn.

Signed: _____Date: _____
Witness: _____Date: _____

"Our deepest fear is not that we are inadequate.
Our deepest fear is that we are powerful beyond measure.
It is our light, not our darkness that frightens us.
We ask ourselves, "Who am I to be brilliant, gorgeous, talented and fabulous?"
Actually, who are you not to be?
You are a child of God.
Your playing small doesn't serve the world.
There's nothing enlightened about shrinking so that other people won't feel insecure around you.
You were born to make manifest the glory of God that is within us.
It's not just in some of us,
it is in everyone.
And as we let our own light shine,
we unconsciously give others the permission to do the same.
As we are liberated from our fear, our presence automatically liberates others."

-Marianne Williamson
Return To Love

Book Suggestion List

Here is a list of books which have helped me along my path of healing. All of them were helpful in awakening a new, stronger part of my self.

Estella, Mary. <u>Natural Foods Cookbook.</u> Tokyo and New York: Japan
    Publications, 1985.

Gates, Donna. <u>The Body Ecology Diet.</u> Atlanta: B.E.D. Publications, 1996.

Huber, Cheri. <u>There Is Nothing Wrong With You.</u> Canada: Keep it Simple Books, 1993.

Northrup, Christina. <u>Women's Bodies, Women's Wisdom.</u> New York: Bantam Books,
    1994.

Pitchford, Paul. <u>Healing with Whole Foods.</u> Berkeley: North Atlantic Books, 1993.

Stevenson, Cloo. <u>Life Revisions.</u> North Carolina: Kidsrights, 1995.

Turner, Kristina. <u>The Self-Healing Cookbook.</u> United States: Earthtones
    Press, 1987.

Swami Paramatmananda Puri. <u>On the Road To Freedom.</u> Mother's Books. (available at
    ammachi.org)

Film Suggestions

<u>Anne of Green Gables</u>. Dir. Kevin Sullivan. With Megan Follows. Sullivan Films,
    1980's.

<u>Anne of Avonlea</u>. Dir. Kevin Sullivan. With Megan Follows. Sullivan Films, 1980's.

Printed in the United States
By Bookmasters